T0355288

Praise for *Veggie Smarts*

"*Veggie Smarts* magically weaves humor, passion, farming, and medicine into a creative package that leaves you searching up new recipe ideas while simultaneously feeling inspired to write poetry. Seriously—read this to learn about how to love and cook vibrant, diverse vegetables. Or read it to better understand the beautiful role each family of veggies plays in our health. You might find yourself dreaming of how you, too, can grow a garden and find joy, healing, and inspiration along the journey. Vegetable Nerds, unite!"

–Jaclyn Lewis Albin, M.D., C.C.M.S., Dip.A.B.L.M.,
Mom, Physician, Culinary and Lifestyle Medicine Specialist,
and Backyard Gardener

"Dr. Michael Compton's *Veggie Smarts* is a delightful and memorable book. Vegetable novices and seasoned veggie professionals alike will gain new insights and inspiration on how to incorporate a wider variety of vegetables into their diets to optimize physical and mental health. I am left inspired to plan meals around 'eight on my plate' and to start a garden to supplement my supermarket vegetable selection. This is an excellent book for both patients and healthcare professionals."

–Jonathan Burgess, M.D., M.P.H., Clinical Assistant Professor,
Lifestyle Psychiatry Clinic, Department of Psychiatry and
Behavioral Sciences, Stanford University School of Medicine

"Getting smarter about vegetables—so highly diverse but from just a few plant families—offers us a way to promote health, reduce risk for (and even reverse) diseases, and support longevity. *Veggie Smarts*, written by a preventionist, lifestyle medicine physician, and organic vegetable farmer, explains our veggies, shares insights from both nutritional science and farming, provides 'free health advice,' and gives poignant, engaging, and humorous confessions of a doctor turned farmer. *Veggie Smarts* is a must-read for anyone who wants to be healthier, happier, and more satisfied with their food, and who wants to be inspired by the possible!"

–Erica Frank, M.D., M.P.H., F.A.C.P.M., Professor,
Faculty of Medicine, University of British Columbia,
Inventor/Founder, www.NextGenU.org

"Vegetables are a vital part of our diet, but many people do not understand them well enough. *Veggie Smarts* explains our vegetables from the perspective of a lifestyle medicine physician and organic vegetable farmer. I highly recommend this essential book—packed full of vitamins, minerals, vegetable stories, and poignant and humorous confessions of a doctor turned farmer. *Veggie Smarts* is a must-read for lifestyle medicine clinicians, for their clients, and for everyone because eating vegetables is important for health."

–Beth Frates, M.D., Associate Professor, Part-Time at
Harvard Medical School and President of the American College
of Lifestyle Medicine

"A refreshing book on vegetables and the pleasures of growing and enjoying them fresh from the garden. Dr. Compton's personal style and welcoming tone provide an excellent book to savor all year—in winter when dreaming of a garden and in summer while raising and eating healthy vegetables."

–**Frederic B. Mayo,** Former Dean of the Faculty at The Culinary Institute of America

"*I should eat more vegetables*. Many of us have had that thought, but when it occurred to physician farmer Michael Compton, a fellow expert in Lifestyle Medicine, it fueled a deep yet engaging journey into eight different families of vegetables, their health benefits, and history. *Veggie Smarts* will inform and delight the reader with compelling stories and interesting details of the bounties of farm and garden, inspiring them to bring plant diversity to their diet...a vital step on the road toward optimal health."

–**Brad B. Moore, M.D., M.P.H., F.A.C.P., Dip.A.B.L.M.,** Director of Lifestyle Medicine, Associate Professor of Medicine, The George Washington University School of Medicine and Health Sciences

"As the former Executive Director for the Hunter College NYC Food Policy Center, with extensive experience with agriculture, food, nutrition, and health programs, I can attest to the importance of people getting smart about vegetables. Dr. Michael Compton's *Veggie Smarts* is an essential read for all practitioners in the agriculture, food, nutrition, and health space—bringing indispensable information to all of us who care about eating sustainably—for the sake of people and the planet."

–**Annette Nielsen,** Journalist

"In this illuminating, vegetable-packed journey, Dr. Compton not only shares how his passion for farming revealed the health benefits of putting eight families of plants on your plate, but also how doing so can be a delicious way to enhance our overall well-being and the world around us. Intertwining nutritional wisdom and its impact on lifestyle medicine with his mid-life foray into small organic farming and practical recipe ideas, *Veggies Smarts* is a must-read for anyone interested in discovering the power and joy of primarily plant-based eating."

–Douglas Noordsy, M.D., Clinical Professor and Director of Lifestyle & Sports Psychiatry Initiative, Associate Director of Stanford Lifestyle Medicine, Stanford University School of Medicine

"*Veggie Smarts* is a thoughtful blend of farming wisdom and nutritional insight. Dr. Compton brings vegetables to life, not only through his expertise as a farmer but with his deep understanding of the health benefits they offer. This book is an essential guide for anyone looking to optimize their diet through the power of diverse, plant-focused nutrition."

–Heather Seid, D.C.N., R.D.N., Program Manager, Bionutrition Research Core at Columbia University's Irving Institute for Clinical and Translational Research

"Michael Compton's wonderful book clearly explains why eating a diverse, plant-based diet is good for you and the planet. It is also a lovely narrative about how an academic doctor became a devoted farmer."

–Laura Sorkin, Author of *Vegetables: The Ultimate Cookbook* Featuring 300+ Delicious Plant-Based Recipes

"Vegetable nerds, Rejoice! As a passionate gardener, I too, have cried over unexpected 'losses' in my home garden, and been astounded by the wonders of old recipes like leek omelet reborn from super fresh ingredients. This book is an ode to transitioning from home gardener to farmer, tracing history, a few recipes along the way, and improving well-being from the power of rediscovering vegetables."

–Julie C. Suarez, Associate Dean for Land Grant Affairs, Cornell University, College of Agriculture and Life Sciences

"Dr. Michael Compton teaches us how to have 'veggie smarts' when it comes to tapping into the power of vegetables in our diets for improving our health and wellbeing."

–John Westerdahl, Ph.D., M.P.H., R.D.N., F.A.N.D., Dip.A.B.L.M., Plant-Based Registered Dietitian Nutritionist, Radio Talk Show Host, *Health & Longevity*–LifeTalk Radio Network

VEGGIE SMARTS

A Doctor and Farmer Grows and Savors
Eight Families of Vegetables

MICHAEL T. COMPTON, M.D., M.P.H.

A REGALO PRESS BOOK
ISBN: 979-8-88845-840-2
ISBN (eBook): 979-8-88845-841-9

Veggie Smarts:
A Doctor and Farmer Grows and Savors Eight Families of Vegetables
© 2025 by Michael T. Compton, M.D., M.P.H.
All Rights Reserved

Cover Design by Jim Villaflores

Publishing Team:
Founder and Publisher – Gretchen Young
Editor—Adriana Senior
Editorial Assistant – Caitlyn Limbaugh
Managing Editor – Aleigha Koss
Production Manager – Alana Mills
Production Editor – Rachel Paul
Associate Production Manager – Kate Harris

This book, as well as any other Regalo Press publications, may be purchased in bulk quantities at a special discounted rate. Contact orders@regalopress.com for more information.

As part of the mission of Regalo Press, a donation is being made to the Hudson Valley CSA Coalition facilitated by Glynwood, as chosen by the author. Find out more about this organization at: https://www. hudsonvalleycsa.org/.

Regalo Press
New York • Nashville
regalopress.com

Published in the United States of America
1 2 3 4 5 6 7 8 9 10

Granny, Essie Mae—
some nights I dream about red currant bushes,
yours and mine, way back then and still today;
and
Granny, Hannah—
some days I daydream about red raspberry canes,
yours and mine, here on this land we've shared.

Contents

A Glossary for Getting *Smart* about *Veggies*

The Brassicas—Brassicaceae

I grow: arugula, bok choy or pak choi, broccoli, green cabbage, red cabbage, savoy cabbage, cauliflower, collards, garlic mustard (a "weed"), horseradish, kale, kohlrabi, land cress, mizuna, mustard greens, napa cabbage, radishes, tatsoi, turnips

Others: broccoli rabe (rapini), broccolini, brussels sprouts, canola, daikon, gai lan, Romanesco, rutabaga, wasabi, watercress

Key Takeaway: In this large family of superfood veggies, the green Brassicas, like broccoli, brussels sprouts, collards, and kale, are densely packed with essential micronutrients such as vitamin C, vitamin K, and folate; health-promoting fiber; and numerous phytonutrients that bolster immune function, support digestive health, and reduce disease risk. Those that are more purple than green—like red cabbage and scarlet kale—contain anthocyanins with antioxidant and anti-inflammatory properties.

The Alliums—Amaryllidaceae

I grow: chives, garlic, leeks, onions, shallots, wild garlic and wild onions ("weeds")

Others: ramps, scallions, walking onions

Key Takeaway: The pungent and delicious—garlicy and oniony—*Allium* bulbs are rich in micronutrients such as vitamin C, vitamin B6, manganese, and selenium, as well as fiber. Their sulfur-containing compounds and other phytonutrients contribute to their immune-, inflammation-, and cardiovascular-related health benefits. Because green veggies are usually more nutritious than white ones, chives and scallions are especially beneficial.

The Legumes—Fabaceae

I grow: bush beans, clover (a "weed"), pea shoots, pole beans, snow peas, yardlong beans

Others: alfalfa sprouts and bean sprouts; edamame, English shelling peas, fava beans, sugar snap peas; dry beans (pulses), including adzuki beans, black beans, black-eyed peas, cannellini beans, chickpeas, cranberry beans, great northern beans, kidney beans, lima beans, lentils, navy beans, pigeon peas, pinto beans, small red beans, small white beans, split peas, and others; peanuts; jicama (a tuber); tamarind

Key Takeaway: The Legumes eaten as sprouts, green pods like snow peas and green beans, and fresh green seeds (like edamame and fava beans) provide an array of micronutrients. Those eaten as dry beans are an excellent source of protein, fiber, and micronutrients, including folate, iron, zinc, and potassium; eaten together with grains (such as beans with rice, hummus and pita, or peanut butter on whole-grain bread), they are a complete protein.

The Chenopods—Amaranthaceae

I grow: beet greens, beets, spinach (perhaps someday), Swiss chard, lamb's quarters and pigweed (superfood "weeds")

Others: amaranth, orach, quinoa

Key Takeaway: The Chenopods are superfoods. Spinach, Swiss chard, and beet tops are all rich in vitamins A, C, and K, as well as minerals like iron, calcium, and potassium, while being packed with antioxidants and fiber. Amaranth and quinoa are two pseudocereals that are a good source of protein, fiber, vitamins A and E, iron, magnesium, and potassium. Lamb's quarters, or "wild spinach," is considered a weed by many but is highly nutritious, as is pigweed.

The Aster Greens—Asteraceae

I grow: catalogna (Italian dandelion), common chicory and dandelion ("weeds"), escarole, frisée (curly endive), lettuce, radicchio, sunflower shoots

Others: artichokes, Belgian endive (witloof), burdock root, cardoon, Jerusalem artichokes (sunchokes), salsify; herbs like chamomile and tarragon

Key Takeaway: The Aster Greens are leafy vegetable greens low in calories and rich in vitamin A, vitamin K, fiber, and minerals like potassium. Variations in color indicate different phytonutrients; for example, deep-purple lettuces and red radicchios contain anthocyanins that are antioxidants and anti-inflammatory compounds.

The Umbellifers—Apiaceae

I grow: carrots, celeriac, celery, cilantro, dill, Florence fennel (finocchio), parsley

Others: lovage; parsnips; herbs including angelica, anise, caraway, chervil, cumin

Key Takeaway: Carrots are rich in vitamin A, vitamin K, and fiber, as well as phytonutrients that support healthy vision, immune function, and skin health. Celery is also nutrient rich and low in calories. The other cousins within the Umbellifers confer health benefits through their own arrays of micronutrients and phytonutrients, as exemplified by phytonutrient-dense Florence fennel.

The Cucurbits—Cucurbitaceae
I grow: cantaloupes, cucumbers, honeydew melons, pattypan squash, pumpkins, yellow squash, watermelons, winter squash, zucchini

Others: bitter melon, calabash, chayote, gourds

Key Takeaway: The Cucurbits are fruits horticulturally, though most are eaten as vegetables culinarily. Cucumbers and summer squash like pattypan, yellow squash, and zucchini are low in calories and rich in vitamin C, vitamin K, potassium, and antioxidants. The skin may be the healthiest part. The Cucurbit fruits are high in water (like juicy, refreshing watermelon) and high in taste but very low in calories.

The Nightshades—Solanaceae
I grow: eggplant, garden huckleberries (or black nightshades), ground cherries, peppers, potatoes, tomatillos, tomatoes

Others: pepinos, sunberries

Key Takeaway: Except for potatoes, which are tubers, the Nightshades are fruits. Tomatoes and peppers offer vitamins A, B6, C, and K, potassium, and phytonutrients like lycopene, which has been linked to eye health, cardiovascular health, and possibly reduced risk of cancer. Tobacco, containing the addictive phytochemical nicotine, is also a Nightshade; though, when smoked, it is obviously highly detrimental to health, compared to the other health-promoting Nightshades.

Vegetables and Herbs from Other Families: asparagus, fiddleheads (from ferns, not flowering plants), ginger, nasturtium, nopal or prickly pear, okra, purslane, rhubarb, sorrel, sweet corn, sweet potatoes, mâche (corn salad or lamb's lettuce), water chestnuts; tubers like cassava (yuca), taro, and yams; and herbs such as anise hyssop, basil, bee balm, bergamot, catnip, lavender, lemon balm, marjoram, mint, oregano, rosemary, sage, savory, and thyme. There are many other vegetables and herbs used in cuisines from cultures outside the United States. And let us not forget mushrooms, which are fungi rather than plants, and seaweed, which is algae, not exactly a plant.

Each of the above-listed vegetables has many cultivated varieties, or cultivars. Sometimes there are dozens of cultivars, as with carrots and winter squash; sometimes hundreds, as with lettuce and peppers; and sometimes thousands, as with potatoes and tomatoes.

1.

How Vegetables Started Growing on Me

I SHOULD EAT MORE VEGETABLES. This has been a recurring thought of mine for years, and it's most likely one of yours. We all know that we should eat more vegetables. It's one of the most doggedly nagging dietary concerns, and, relatedly, health concerns, of so many of us. We should all eat more vegetables. But for whatever reasons, we find it hard to do so, despite doctors, nutritionists, journalists, environmentalists, family, friends, inner voices, and others telling us that we should.

Take carrots, for example. Most of us would secretly, if not openly, acknowledge that we should eat more carrots. But something holds us back, and it's not a lack of carrots. Most of us admit that we eat too little kale, not nearly enough beets, and a glaringly insufficient amount of Swiss chard, if we eat any Swiss chard at all.

As a farmer, though not a botanist, I know how to grow plants—even if I know little about the intricate anatomy of a flower, or exactly how photosynthesis works, or why roots know to grow down and stems to grow up. As a doctor, though not a dietitian, I know that eating diverse vegetables across a number of families of plants is health promoting, even if I know little about exactly why vitamin A is good for our eyes or specifically how much manganese and magnesium we should be striving for.

College, medical school, and specialty training in psychiatry, preventive medicine, and lifestyle medicine had taken this proverbial boy off the farm, but as all who know the old saying might suspect, the farm had not been taken out of me. A midlife rejuvenation—some might call it a midlife crisis—was bound to happen, and this boy from a farm, turned doctor and expert on disease prevention and nutrition, built himself a farm. As my little farm has been growing, I've become intimately familiar with a multitude of vegetables across eight families, and I want to share what I've learned. I've also been arriving at a simple rule of thumb on how I can best improve my health, and increase my happiness, by optimizing what and how I eat: eating veggies smartly. The first of our eight families will be the Brassicaceae, also known as the cabbage or mustard family—or, as I've called it, the "Brassicas"—but let's start by thinking about carrots.

I NOW EAT CARROTS

Most of us know about the animals that are eaten in the form of pork, beef, foul, fish, shellfish, and so on. We all also have a good understanding of dairy (like milk, cream, butter, yogurt, and the myriad cheeses), eggs, and even the various grains, from oatmeal to rice to lots of wheat flour. My focus is eight families of plants that we should all know very well from top to bottom.

Before we embark on understanding and eating these families of plants, one at a time, across eight chapters, I'd like for you to first think about your relationship to just four vegetables in a simple thought exercise. And I'll tell you about my relationship to them, how it has changed, and how I'm now healthier and happier for it.

First, carrots.

Do you like carrots? Stop and really think about it. What is your relationship with carrots? I know it's a strange thing for a psychiatrist to ask.

Do you buy carrots at the grocery store? If so, do you get them bundled with stems and leaves on top, or bagged without the green parts? If bagged, are they whole or shredded down to "baby" carrots? Do you order carrots as a side in restaurants? Or do any of your favorite restaurants not offer carrots as a side? Imagine the taste of carrots, and any related associations, from childhood or adulthood. How do you feel about eating carrots?

I personally was never a fan of carrots. In fact, I really found no reason to eat them, other than knowing that I was supposed to eat them. We are all supposed to because everyone knows that they're good for us. Something about the beta-carotene, which the body converts to vitamin A—or retinol—being good for your eyes. Doctors and nutritionists say that we should eat carrots. I never really cared for carrots, though, even as a doctor. But now carrots are part of how I eat year-round. I pull the last carrots after the ground has frozen and thawed several times, in November, and they store well all the way through fall and winter, nearly until spring, when I begin pulling the first carrots in late June.

More on carrots later, including my favorite: honey roasted carrots, which I consider to be ambrosia.

Now think about celery. How much do you like celery? Do you buy it in the grocery store? Ever see it at restaurants, aside from its being used to add some crunch alongside buffalo wings? How do you feel about eating celery? Do you crave it? Avoid it? Are you ambivalent toward it?

Again, I personally never saw a real need for celery and never had much interest in it. Especially raw. I thought it too stringy, with a distinct, strong, and not necessarily pleasant taste, and seemingly only useful to add some interesting texture to chicken salad and tuna salad. But now, celery has become one of my biggest summer delights, especially given that I consider it to be the fussiest of all the vegetables on my farm. I've had a long journey with celery, from rooftop planters in our nation's capital to an excess on the farm needing to be harvested and requiring signs at the farmers markets advising "last week for celery." I now savor—dare I say crave—fresh-cut celery. Celery makes me happy. And not just the stalks but also the celery leaves, which can transform an otherwise regular entrée into cuisine. Little had I known, just a few years ago, that celery is foundational to many of the world's greatest soups.

Next, fennel—Florence fennel. You know, the big white bulbs with the anise or licorice smell and taste. What is your relationship to fennel? Do you cook with it? Any favorite recipes? Do you add it to salads? If you come from an Italian heritage, I'm talking about finocchio, and your answer will likely be quite different from that of those of us with no Italian roots.

Growing up and throughout my young adulthood, I had never eaten fennel. I felt that since I had strongly disliked the taste of licorice as a child, I would have no interest in eating fennel in any way, shape, or form. Ever. In fact, I don't recall having ever eaten it intentionally; though perhaps it was stealthily hidden in some crunchy, healthy first-course salad in an upscale restaurant when my partner Ken and I lived in Washington, DC, or New York City. But now, given the enthusiasm for fennel among many of my CSA (community supported agriculture, or farm share) members and farmers market customers, it's been growing on me. I love growing it; thus, I now love eating it. With my new vantage point as an organic farmer, loving these beautiful plants, I wonder why fresh, local, springtime fennel isn't an essential, even if small, part of what we all eat.

Finally, parsley. When you hear "parsley," do you think of the curly variety or the flat-leaf Italian type? When do you eat it? How do you eat it—freshly chopped, or dried as a spice? How much of both of those, fresh herb or dried spice, do you like to use when a recipe calls for a pinch or a smidgeon, or as a garnish? Imagine the smell of fresh parsley, the taste, the texture. Which of your favorite dishes always have parsley?

For me, of course I had eaten plenty of parsley. I had always viewed it as a garnish and never thought much about it. Now with the perspective of a parsley grower, or even a parsley-growing enthusiast, I've elevated it from an herb by the tablespoon to a vegetable by the handful. I use it especially for my favorite pesto. I'll give you the recipe.

I begin this vegetable journey with these four vegetables because they have grown on me as I have been growing them. In building a compact, highly diversified organic farm, these four vegetables were necessities. Any respectable farmers market stand has beautiful bunches of carrots in both spring and fall. And a CSA that boasts "gourmet" produce must have Florence fennel and both curly parsley and flat Italian parsley. And, yes, I grow celery, which, despite being at the top of my list of high-maintenance, finicky plants, is an annual favorite.

Throughout this book, I encourage you to think in this same way about each of the vegetables to be named. And for those you're less familiar with, I encourage you to seek them out and give them a try. For your health and your happiness.

I NOW EAT CARROTS, CELERY, FENNEL, AND PARSLEY

Growing and savoring carrots, celery, fennel, and parsley has been an adventure. I don't recall our garden growing up, or Granny's, boasting any of these pretty plants. Perhaps that's why I never saw much use for them until adulthood, until I started growing them.

I now eat all four of these vegetables regularly, and I savor them. I feel a sense of excitement in pulling a handful of carrots out of the ground—never knowing what to expect and always feeling delighted, and sometimes surprised, in the shapes and sizes that are revealed. (Not only is it magic to me, but kids really think it's magic, always making them giggle and want to take a bite.) When early summer celery is ready to be cut, I might appear a bit fanatical about it. And every spring, I can't resist taking and sharing pictures of my stand of Florence fennel, since it's such a pretty and stately sight. Most importantly, though, these four vegetables have grown on me because they make me healthy. As part of *eight on my plate*, I strive to eat one of these *cousins* every day. Some days I succeed; some days I don't.

So how are these seemingly very different four vegetables—carrots, celery, fennel, and parsley—alike? Why did I pick them for this simple thought exercise?

They are all cousins in a wonderful family of flowering plants called the Apiaceae, or Umbelliferae: the Umbellifers. They seem so different (like carrots compared to parsley) because humans have identified and selectively grown specific attributes within the family members that serve us well culinarily and nutritionally. Though they're all part of one big extended family, we eat different parts of Apiaceae plants. The carrot, of course, is a root, like another cousin in this family, the parsnip. As for celery, we eat the long stems. And a fennel bulb is the lowest portion of the stem that becomes swollen and layered. Obviously, parsley is grown neither for its roots nor for its stems but for its leaves. The Umbellifers are a family of plants that provide us with tremendous nutritional value, some of which is shared across the family, and some portion quite specific to the individual Umbellifer cousins. I strive to eat at least one Umbellifer vegetable each day.

A COW THAT ONLY FEELS GOOD SOMETIMES

After that brief Umbellifer getting-to-know-you, let's take a plant-nerd taxonomy tangent. Its relevance to *eight on my plate* will soon become apparent. Taxonomy groups plants by shared characteristics, like the beautiful, lacy, umbrella-like flowers shared by the Umbellifer cousins. Knowing *family*, *genus*, and *species* is important on the farm for understanding life cycle, planning crop rotations, and preparing for the most likely pests. But it can also be important in eating the healthiest of meals.

In high school biology, you might have learned that "King Phillip Came Over From Great Spain," or "King Phillip Cried Out For Good Soup." Or for those of us growing up in the country, where kings and Spain seemed way too foreign, it was: "Kevin's Poor Cow Only Feels Good Sometimes." That's the one I memorized, as it seemed so close to home—my older brother Kevin did, in fact, tend to some ailing Holsteins on the dairy farm we lived on. Whatever the mnemonic device used in the classroom, which you may or may not have set into your long-term memory, the goal was this: Kingdom, Phylum, Class, Order, Family, Genus, Species.

The plant kingdom is obviously very different from the animal kingdom. Plants are distinguished from animals by a number of traits; for example, they exhibit sedentary growth—basically meaning that they have stems instead of legs. And whereas animals (including ourselves and our cats and dogs) have to eat organic molecules, plants are able to use sunlight to synthesize their own food (and ours) from carbon dioxide (in the air) and water. Sunshine plus air plus rain. That's *photosynthesis*, which is some amazingly cool biology, especially since it gives us much-needed oxygen as a byproduct.

The plant kingdom is first divided into seven to fourteen phyla, or divisions, depending on whom you're reading and when they were writing. These phyla or divisions include the Bryophyta, or the mosses; Pteridophyta, the ferns; and Coniferophyta, the conifers like pine trees, and so on. Here, throughout, I deal exclusively with the single phylum of Magnoliophyta, or Angiospermae: the flowering plants. And among the more than four hundred families of flowering plants, I'll cover just a few genera and species from just eight families, all of which have come to be our veggies.

Back to taxonomy, the basic unit of classification is a *species*, a group able to breed among itself, bearing resembling offspring. The broader classification is the *genus*, or, in its plural form, *genera*. Just for fun, I call members of the same genus *siblings*, or brothers and sisters, and family members from different genera *cousins*. As an example, when I eventually make my way to the beloved Solanaceae family, the Nightshades—which includes tomatoes, peppers, and eggplants, among others—the tomato plant is *Solanum lycopersicum*, the pepper plant is *Capsicum annuum*, and the eggplant plant is *Solanum melongena*. As such, I consider tomato and eggplant to be siblings (both in the *Solanum* genus), and peppers to be their spicy cousin. But they're all from the same big family, the Nightshades.

THE TAXONOMY OF A SIMPLE SALAD

The goal of eight on my plate is striving to eat *diverse* vegetables, which is why taxonomy is important, especially in terms of families, genera, and species. Let's take a spring salad as an example.

Merveille des Quatre Saisons is a savoyed (curly leafed) French heirloom butterhead lettuce with contrasting pink, red, light green, and dark green leaves. It's crisp, sweet, and delicious. And it's gorgeous. You'll never find it in a grocery store, as it's far too delicate for long hauls in 18-wheelers. Because it's such a mouthful, on the farm, I call it "MdQS." As we'll see in the Asteraceae chapter (on the Aster Greens), the genus and species of MdQS, like every other lettuce, is *Lactuca sativa*. All lettuces are not just siblings, but are fraternal twins, so to speak.

Atop the lightly dressed butterhead—MdQS—I'll add some sliced celery, the genus and species of which is *Apium graveolens*, within, as you know, the Apiaceae family, or the Umbellifers. One more topping on this simple, sweet lettuce salad is a sliced French breakfast radish, among many varieties of radish, within the Brassicaceae family, or the Brassicas.

It's a simple salad that I've assembled. But it includes plants from three families. The Aster Greens (the lettuce), the Umbellifers (the celery), and the Brassicas (the radish). As such, this salad gives us an array of micronutrients (vitamins and minerals) like vitamins A, C, and K, along with copper, manganese, and potassium—much more than a simple Asteraceae-only Caesar with just romaine lettuce would. And more than a salad of mixed lettuces, frisée, and radicchio would, because they are all from one family, the Aster

Greens. Eating healthy is about combining vegetables across multiple families. And it's not hard, because we're generally dealing with veggies from only eight. This simple, tasty, and healthy salad has three. Adding a ripe, juicy, delicious, sliced Campari tomato come late July would make it four, a few cut green beans would make it five, and so on. The more of the eight families it has, the healthier the meal will be.

One straightforward way to strive for, or achieve, a highly diversified, mostly plant-based way of eating is to count the vegetable families appearing on one's plate at a meal and over the course of one's combined daily meals. Since the vast majority of our vegetables come from just eight families, eight on my plate is a simple approach of counting not just the vegetables but also the families in which they are situated. I've eaten especially healthily when I've achieved eight on my plate—at least one Brassica, at least one Allium, at least one Legume, at least one Chenopod, at least one Umbellifer, at least one Aster Green, at least one Cucurbit, and at least one Nightshade—all in a day. If these families' surnames are hard to remember, create a mnemonic for yourself, perhaps something like: "Nutrition And Longevity Attained By Creating Unique Cuisine" (Nightshades, Alliums, Legumes, Aster Greens, Brassicas, Chenopods, Umbellifers, Cucurbits); or "Nutrition And Longevity Attained By Chopping Up Chard"; or one of your own.

AN UNAPOLOGETIC VEGETABLE SNOB, A VEGETABLE BON VIVANT

As a farm boy who grew into a midlife farm nerd, I've really gotten to know these vegetable plants, like from a tiny, round seed sown in a flat under a quarter inch of home-made seed-starting mix in the greenhouse on March 20 to a gorgeous and delicious head of Savoy cabbage two and a half months later. My interest and enthusiasm in growing these vegetables is the source of my interest in healthy eating. I've become the particular type of foodie that I refer to as a "vegetable snob," meaning I seek out the best and poo-poo iceberg lettuce, bell peppers, and the like. You can call me a snob. Or you can join me.

Small, local "market farms" and community supported agriculture (CSA) farms like mine allow one to embrace this way of eating because they usually strive to grow as many vegetables as possible—and in many cases, many cultivars (cultivated varieties) of many of those vegetables. That's because our goal is to provide our customers with *all* their vegetables across the entire growing season. Dairy farms focus on milk, berry farms focus on berries, and market and CSA farms focus on growing the full array of veggies for their dedicated customers. CSA members expect diversity across the twenty or more weeks of receiving farm shares. Ironically, larger farms grow fewer species, and the very largest farms usually grow only one, perhaps rotating with a second (think field corn and soybeans, virtually all of which, as I'll explain, nowadays are genetically modified organisms, or GMOs, used in our ketchup and mayonnaise and the like). Buying from small, local farms at farm stands and farmers markets—or joining one as a CSA member—ensures that you'll get a bounty of seasonal vegetables at their peak of freshness, produced in a way that's good for our soil, our water, and the environment in general.

Small, local farms take pride in growing many varieties of nearly all the vegetables. For example, as I'll detail when I get to the Aster Greens, I typically grow eight or nine types of lettuce. There might only be three or four options in even the largest of supermarkets, one of which, soapbox pending, doesn't even really count as lettuce, in my view.

Only several dozen of the countless vegetable cultivars are available in grocery stores, supermarkets, and the food distributors that supply most restaurants. As such, those are the ones we tend to eat. Among those several dozen varieties, most of us have settled on a few by habit, based on how much time we want to spend in the kitchen (or not), what we ate and did not eat growing up, and how our eating habits have been shaped within our family or among our friends. The specific several dozen varieties that we find in the grocery store are there largely because of their cultural properties (such as how easy or hard they are for farmers to grow, harvest, and transport on a mass scale), their appearance (like those giant, perfect bell peppers), and their ease of use in the kitchen (as in those large, perfectly round, uniform slicing tomatoes, as compared to ribbed and wrinkled, funny-shaped heirloom tomatoes).

The limited array of grocery store produce includes those big, beautiful green, yellow, orange, and red bell peppers, the perfect red(ish) slicing tomatoes, the alarmingly long English cucumbers wrapped tightly in thick plastic to prevent any blemish, and the yellow onions that all seem identical in size. I used to think of these as staples in the kitchen. Since becoming a farmer, though, they seem to be novelties, even peculiarities. Yes, I'm a vegetable snob.

On the farm, I grow eight varieties of peppers each year, none of which are bell peppers. The heirloom tomatoes are rarely perfect in appearance, though they're splendid in taste. The cucumbers are not wrapped in plastic, and the onions come in different sizes.

Some of my vegetables are drop-dead gorgeous varieties that are completely missing in the grocery store, like MdQS, petit Marseillais peppers, green zebra tomatoes, and the rainbow blend of colorful carrots. Either their shelf life is too short, their cultivation is too difficult for larger-scale production, or customers are too unaccustomed to their looks for the grocery store to stock them. That's the beauty of CSA farm shares and farmers markets—the beauty of *diversity*.

The vegetables we'll explore here have grown on me because I've been growing them. Growing them year after year has taught me about their seeds, their germination preferences, how they like to be tended to, what makes them more generous, and what their greatest struggles are.

As is obvious, our focus here is on just eight families, though there are vegetables that come from a few other families that I'll describe as "one-hit wonders," like asparagus, okra, and sweet potatoes. The vegetables that we'll consider are only a few species within a few genera of our eight families (from among more than four hundred) of flowering plants. Of all the plants on earth, we eat only a very, very small number of them, which is further reason why we should have veggie smarts and know them very well.

There is actually no real reason why we don't eat many more plants as veggies, both within and outside of the eight families. It has just become a matter of convenience, tradition, availability, and habit to rely on the several dozen that we do eat. I'll occasionally mention eating certain weeds. Yes, eating weeds, which could be seen as a delicacy, since they're completely impossible to find in the grocery store, and given the dearth of really good recipes for superfood weeds like clover, purslane, garlic mustard, lamb's quarters, pigweed, and the like.

While I do tout myself, sarcastically and sassily, as an unapologetic vegetable snob, the more appropriate appellation would be a vegetable bon vivant. In perfecting my pastime—growing vegetables for myself and my partner, then for neighbors, and eventually for CSA farm share members and farmers market customers—I found myself eating, enthusiastically savoring, in fact, the very vegetables I was evidently so good at growing. I became a vegetable aficionado. A vegetable connoisseur. A vegetable enthusiast. Eating so well, so healthily and happily—savoring these plants, socializing around my homegrown gourmet produce, from arugula to zucchini—I found myself becoming a vegetable bon vivant, living the good life, with these sixty or so vegetables across about ninety varieties to which I so carefully tend. My journey is that of a nerdy doctor having a highly productive midlife crisis by becoming a very nerdy farmer—one who came to realize that all these vegetables fit into eight families of plants, each with their own constellation of health-promoting micronutrients and phytochemicals (the latter also called phytonutrients: carotenoids like beta-carotene and lycopene, flavonoids like quercetin and kaempferol, sulfur-containing compounds, and others that would undoubtedly make me healthier, happier, and live longer). The good life.

VEGGIE SMARTS

Our country has an eating problem—a big eating problem. In its 2020–2025 *Dietary Guidelines* documentation, the US federal government tells us that 74 percent of American adults are overweight or obese. Closely related to that figure, 75 percent have eating patterns low in vegetables and fruits, and 77 percent exceed the recommended limit for saturated fat, meaning animal fats like meats, eggs, butter, and all that wonderful cheese. Over the past fifteen years, our average Healthy Eating Index score has varied little, bouncing around between fifty-six and sixty (out of one hundred points), and, thus, not surprisingly, six out of ten American adults are living with one or more food-related chronic diseases. Six out of ten. Given these statistics, we all need to get smart about veggies.

What you'll discover in these pages—as you gain veggie smarts and consider the eight-on-my-plate way of eating—holds promise to lower your risk of being overweight, of prediabetes and type 2 diabetes, of heart disease, of cancer, and probably of depression and addictions (except for a few veggie addictions, which I'll encourage). And if you already have any of those conditions, eight on my plate should be at the center of your treatment, with a goal of disease reversal. Getting smart about eating vegetables can also increase your likelihood of a really long life, since heart disease and cancer are, by far, our leading causes of death.

I write as a doctor who got smart about vegetables by being a farmer. Even with many hours of physiology and pathophysiology in medical school, we learned next to nothing about what we should eat for ideal health, or how we should eat, for all of us now and in the future. We learned virtually nothing about vegetables, except, as I'll describe, the physiology behind bean flatulence, that beets can mimic blood in the urine, and that potatoes have a relatively high glycemic index, which is of relevance to diabetes. This, despite having heard the adage that food is medicine, or, more specifically, "Let food be thy medicine and medicine be thy food," as said Hippocrates, the father of medicine whose oath we medical doctors continue to take more than 2,400 years after his practice. It was a quarter of a century after taking the oath that I finally came to understand what Hippocrates really meant.

I got smart about vegetables by growing them. I needed to understand their seeds, their seedlings, how they grow, and exactly when to harvest them so that I could best serve my farm customers. And with so much produce around— bushel-baskets full, wheelbarrows full, a farmers market delivery van full, and a kitchen full—I needed to get smart about how to eat them. So, I got veggie smarts, and I hope to share them with you.

What does *veggie smarts* really mean? Here's my definition, though it doesn't appear in the Oxford English Dictionary or Webster's. Yet.

Veggie smarts means having a thorough understanding of vegetables so that meals will be more delicious and health will be optimized. It means knowing how the different vegetables are and are not related to one another, thereby enhancing selections for a highly diversified, mostly plant-based way of eating that promotes physical and mental health and prevents or reverses poor health and disease. It is the ability to confidently find, understand, and eat vegetables smartly, all the while cultivating curiosity about how vegetables are grown on farms and can be grown at home. A botanical understanding of these families brings about a culinary understanding of them, which benefits one's food choices and, thus, one's health. Having veggie smarts informs decisions and actions at grocery stores and other places where vegetables are purchased, in restaurants, in the home garden, in the kitchen, and around the table. Having veggie smarts is about vegetable knowledge, but it is also a mindset and a commitment to oneself. My hypothesis, admittedly entirely untested, is that understanding our veggies better is conducive to eating more of them. It sure worked for me.

I start my dinner most nights with a salad, and I try to plan the salad, family-wise, around the entrée and/or vegetables that are to be served, whether at home or in a restaurant, to increase the number of families I'll be eating. If roasted broccoli is coming up, for example, I'd never start with an arugula, kale, or watercress salad (all Brassicas like the broccoli), but a spinach or lettuce salad would be perfect. If white beans with escarole are to be served, I'd never start with a green bean or radicchio salad, but a kale Caesar would be perfect. If the baked cod entrée comes with a side of Swiss chard (which I hope it does), I'd never start with a spinach salad, but a radicchio salad is just right. I use the same process to select sides of vegetables. It's about eating eight families. And that's why we need to learn about those eight families.

Throughout this book, in addition to telling some stories about my farm and my farmhouse, I aim to impart upon you veggie smarts. As I move through the families, I won't have much to say about macronutrients: the carbohydrates, proteins, and fats that provide us with the large quantities of key elements we need (carbon, hydrogen, nitrogen, oxygen, phosphorus, sulfur, calcium, sodium, potassium, magnesium, and chloride). The bottom line is that a whole-foods, plant-predominant eating pattern that is *diverse*—well-prepared vegetables across multiple families, genera, and species—will give us everything we need in terms of carbohydrates, proteins, and fats. Since all vegetables are low in fat, I'm not going to say much more about fat at all. In fact, one of the liberating aspects of a whole-foods, plant-predominant eating pattern is that you can stop worrying about fat and protein and carbohydrates altogether. No more concern about getting enough protein or eating too much fat. Relatedly, eating enough raw and minimally processed vegetables is certain to give us ample disease-fighting fiber. With eight on my plate, you can check that box, too, never needing to give fiber another thought.

While I'll give some basic details about micronutrients (vitamins and minerals) and a few of the phytonutrients, those aren't a main concern; what really matters is that we eat vegetables across all eight families, ideally daily. A meal with four families is good. One with five is better. One with six is bordering on extreme. One with seven is exceedingly healthy. One with eight is outrageously health promoting. I challenge myself to eat as many of the eight families per meal—or across the day—as possible.

The very basic recipes I provide show my simple approach to eating vegetables that I gathered directly from the gardens or that were left over after the week's farmers markets. They rely on few ingredients and are farmer inspired rather than chef inspired, showing how I eat the very plants that I spent so many hours nurturing. The goal is to build the habit of eating the full diversity of vegetables in straightforward ways before moving on to more complex and challenging recipes. Amazing vegetable cookbooks exist, and I encourage you to seek them out as part of your journey toward mastering veggie smarts.

2.

How I Started Growing Vegetables

DURING A NUMBER OF HAPPY YEARS in training and my early career in psychiatry, preventive medicine, and public health at Emory University in Atlanta, Ken and I renovated a late 1940s little brick house and then built a brand-new Craftsman bungalow on the open lot next door. We lived in a post–World War II–era bungalow neighborhood called Jefferson Park on the south side of town—in East Point (South Point, in my mind, would have seemed a more appropriate name). The "old" house required much interior work, but it was the outside work of redesigning the landscaping that appealed most to me.

The builder's blueprints for the new house we had built included details of the landscaping, and the job would be done by professionals, as my career was keeping me increasingly busy. The backyard drawings boasted, much to my curiosity and delight, three raised beds of four feet by four feet each. It had been the builder's idea, not my own. He was not aware of my childhood in flower patches and vegetable gardens, and I had mostly given up that part of my life long ago. I was excited to see those raised beds on his drawings, though, as it gave me the intriguing idea that perhaps I could grow a few vegetables—something I hadn't thought to do since my elementary and middle school years, before academics had taken over most of my waking hours.

In those little raised beds—rich, nutritious soil bounded by heavy timbers—I grew mostly herbs, though I occasionally grew a tomato plant or zucchini plant. It was not a productive enough operation to consider myself as really growing any substantial vegetables, but it made the backyard look pretty: mostly manicured, but with some veggies growing, harkening back to days of eating homegrown food. Perhaps Granny would have been proud of me.

After all, my green thumbs had come primarily from Granny, who had always lived next door when I was growing up. Learning to grow and eat vegetables started at an early age, in southwestern Virginia. We had a big garden each year, replete with green beans, October beans, sweet corn, tomatoes, and potatoes that we would can, freeze, and store. I learned about these various activities and hard work alongside my father, mother, brother, and two sisters and in close proximity to a multitude of aunts, uncles, cousins, and their gardens. Granny's garden, which I remember as an extension of our own, creating one long vegetable plot crossing our respective backyards, always seemed the most bountiful. And beyond the vegetable garden, her yard had some special delights that made forever impressions on my tastebuds, especially the few vines of Concord grapes, the single red currant bush, and the pear and cherry trees scattered across the landscape.

There were also flowers all around her house, like the big, beautiful, fragrant purple bearded irises I came to love so much that before advancing past elementary school, I felt a strong need to have my own flower garden where I could grow snapdragons and zinnias, among others. The plow-up to create my flower garden was a pretty straightforward job, since we lived on a dairy farm where my father could easily connect a plow to a tractor and turn sod into soil, which he did for me one evening after tending to and milking the Holsteins.

Ken's and my new house in Atlanta would not have a large garden like those I had growing up, but the builder's idea definitely reawakened green thumbs that Granny might have thought at the time that I had turned in for a white collar. The amount of energy I expended on those three little raised beds didn't yield very much in the form of food, but I nonetheless felt proud when friends were dining with us and the tomato and basil were "fresh from Michael's garden."

MARTINIS, ALONG WITH CELERY AND PEANUT BUTTER

After nearly fifteen years in Atlanta, Ken and I decided to shake things up and make a move to Washington, DC, where I had wanted to live since attending college in Fredericksburg, just over an hour south of the capital. George Washington University's medical school would be my professional home for the next three years, and they were great ones. We gave up both vehicles, making the capital city a truly ambulatory experience. I had a 1.2-mile walk to work each day, through Logan Circle, then Dupont Circle, and finally to Foggy Bottom. I continued to immerse myself in psychiatric research, and my career advanced commendably. I spent no time thinking about vegetables, except, perhaps when deciding between the iceberg or the romaine, or the giant yellow bell pepper or the giant red one, in the grocery store.

In those days, I never gave much thought to farm-fresh, local produce. I shopped at grocery stores, and we ate out way too much. Yet, I was magnetically pulled to the farmers market in Dupont Circle on Sunday mornings, unsure why the tables of honey, homemade hot sauces, little baskets of cherry tomatoes, and freshly pulled carrots seemed so magical to me. It was like a weekly trip to the proverbial candy shop, even if most such trips resulted only in a blueberry muffin, made by a farmer with actual blueberries, or a few apples for the week. I felt drawn to the farmers' stands, embarrassingly staring at the gorgeous and colorful produce, not even consciously connecting it to Granny or my childhood replete with produce and flowers.

During our stint in DC, both our initial apartment in Dupont Circle and then a newly redone condominium in an old brick townhouse in Logan Circle shared one feature in common: a rooftop deck. That uncommon amenity was not coincidental; I think Ken and I both felt that we required a rooftop deck, partly to have an interesting urban view of other rooftops, as well as a tiny sliver of the Washington Monument, and partly so that we would have a private place to make vitamin D. For me, though, that first rooftop requirement came with another: planters for growing some flowers and maybe a few vegetables, since we didn't have a yard for it.

One year at the springtime farmers market in Dupont Circle, I came across some young celery plants. I'm not sure that I had ever seen four packs of celery. I now know that young celery plants are incredibly hard to come by, and I understand that's because they are fussy and finicky to grow. But I became determined to grow celery, despite having no plans to ever eat it, because it was not something we grew when I was a boy, and I wanted to try something new. I bought the entire tray of young celery plants, figuring that it would make for an unusual and interesting rooftop experience. There were thirty-two of them. Perhaps this was a harbinger of my tendency to grow way too much produce, someday to be fully manifested during my calling and conversion from gardener to farmer.

The rooftop celery experiment happened well before I really got to know the hard part of growing celery—the very slow germination and the flimsy seedlings. These plants in four packs were very well established and grew well in the rooftop planters. It was the only thing I grew up there that year, and it was a lot of celery. I liked to show it off to house guests. Wine or cocktails on the rooftop would be accompanied by a container of ranch dressing and a jar of peanut butter. Crunchy and delicious crudités alongside the Malbec or martinis.

KITCHENS BIG AND SMALL

After three years in our nation's capital, a hard-to-resist career opportunity presented itself in Manhattan. That's right—New York City, a place that had always seemed overdone, overvalued, and overcrowded to me. A stipulation of living in a small Manhattan apartment, for both of us, was having a weekend home in the countryside. And we were able to afford it with my new job. A countryside cottage. A release valve and shock absorber to help survive big city life. A patch of private weekend green space to compensate for the lack of green in our weekday work lives.

When a search on Long Island didn't turn up the exact cottage we were looking for, several friends suggested that we extend our search to the Hudson Valley, a place I had, though I'm now ashamed to admit it, never heard of. But what a beautiful place it turned out to be. A place that would change my life. A place that would revolutionize my way of eating. A place that would turn me into a farmer.

After just a couple of weekends visiting only a few properties—primarily several modernized old stone houses, gems in the Hudson Valley because of its Dutch and French heritage—we found the one. We had focused on old stone houses because I had always been very fond of and intrigued by them; I fancy that my ancestors came from the Cotswolds region of England, though they might well have been from Old Compton Street in London. Now I had my own old stone house, replete with every modern amenity imaginable. And it came with land.

The old stone house was about 185 years old, and the newer additions were from the 1970s (a large living room with vaulted ceilings and an amazing fireplace that replaced a former lean-to shed off the back); 1998 (another large living room beyond the first one, again with vaulted ceilings and surrounded by windows, which had been built by the former owner, Yancey, as her artist's studio); and the mid-2000s (the kitchen on the right side of the stone house and the huge primary suite on the left, also by Yancey). I would soon start referring to our new home—at least the stone portion—as the "Delamater House," because of a one-paragraph history that Yancey had left behind and because it seemed fitting for such an old house to have a formal name.

The property is on the winding Union Center Road in the Town of Esopus, named for the tribe of Lenape whose land this had been. A lot of 9.95 acres (we round up and call it ten) was a lot of land—partly wooded, partly over-grown, but mostly in lawn grass, and much of that bordered by landscaped flower gardens. That was according to the pictures, which we relied on heavily since the property had been under at least six inches of snow each of the several times we visited. It was more than a cottage, and it would be a lot of work to maintain the house and the property. But as it was just a weekend home, we would hire a weekly mower for the summers, a quarterly pond guy, someone to plow the snow from the driveway, and a biweekly housekeeper.

When we signed the closing paperwork in mid-March—while the property *still* remained under snow—we were delighted with the house, especially the very well equipped, large, modern kitchen. Compared to the nearly unusable closet of a kitchen in our Manhattan apartment, this was a *real* kitchen. It was very large, it had everything, and it would become the center of the house, even though the house is really centered around the original old stone building that had been home to many families across many generations. The kitchen would immediately become the place where we would spend much of our time; eventually, it would be a place that would receive countless baskets of fresh produce from what would, within several years, become a small farm operation. And an organic-certified one at that. Although I had no thoughts of growing vegetables when we bought the place, that changed when I discovered something when the snow melted beside the two-car garage just a short way down the driveway: a garden that would call me.

DUTCH WOODEN SHOES, AND TULIPS

We had initiatlly naïvely assumed that the old stone house had been built by Dutch settlers, and on our weekend trips home to the countryside, we set about buying wooden shoes and other Dutch-inspired antiques to add to the décor. In the fall, I planted tulip bulbs to ensure a real Dutch feel for the early springtime. As it turns out, with some research it became apparent that the old stone house had been built by people bearing a French last name, not a Dutch one. We kept the wooden shoes, but the deer ate all the tulips in the springtime. Perhaps they were descended from deer who had known the French-descendent homeowners, telling us, not subtly, that this had not been a Dutch place. I was quick to discover, however, that the deer—an ongoing menace and, at the same time, intrigue on our property—would step over and around daffodils to reach the delectable tulips, not daring to take a bite from the bright white and yellow daffodils. I found it curious because I had always assumed that tulips and daffodils were closely related and thus would taste alike. But that was well before I read up on plant taxonomy and realized that daffodils, among the Amaryllidaceae, probably taste a bit too much like garlic and onions for the deer to find delectable.

As we became curious about the original owners of the old stone house, the first clue, in addition to the paragraph Yancey had left us, was found on a cornerstone on the front porch. An etching reads: "CDBD : HD : IL" (and, underneath the "CDBD : HD," "1828"). The letters represent Cornelius Du Bois Delamater and his wife, Hannah Delamater, presumably carved when the house was built in 1828. The "IL" amendment, as I would eventually figure out—after a lot of research—is from a later owner (Ira Lambert) who thought it appropriate to add his own initials nearly sixty years later. I wouldn't dare add my own, knowing that my stay here is likely short and that others will live and eat in this old stone house without adding theirs. When I looked further into the "IL" addendum, I discovered that Ira was not a farmer like the Delamaters but a merchant or grocery store owner. By the late 1800s, those who were well off didn't have to grow all their own food or barter with neighbors as the Delamaters had. His store likely sold coffee, tea, sugar, flour, and spices.

At thirty-two feet across the front and back and twenty-four feet along the sides, the old stone house is a simple rectangle. With two-feet-thick walls on the sides and 2.5-feet-thick walls on the front and back, this equates to 540 square feet. The entire ground floor is our dining room. Up the steep stairs is a guest bedroom, along with a bathroom and small sitting area. Houses were small back then. Additions were needed over time.

The little history *Esopus* by Karl R. and Susan B. Wick makes the following note about a photograph of the old stone house taken in about 1910, when the house was already more than eighty years old: "It is an older stone house with a wood-framed addition, but the reader should notice the style of the stone. The front of the house is built of cut stone, not fieldstone. This is uncommon on early houses." Cornelius and Hannah had upgraded to a more classic design for the front stonework. The two-story wood addition is long gone, though a shadow of it remains on the left side of the old stone house. Now, multiple additions exist, and the main living quarters—most notably the kitchen that sold us on the place—have little to remind one of the 1800s.

THIS IS YANCEY'S PROPERTY

Her name was Mary Yancey Walker, but, in these parts, everyone knew her as Yancey. And everyone knew her. Our new property, as we would quickly find out, was referred to in these parts as Yancey's property. Yancey bought the old stone house in 1998, when it had just the one addition—the first living room off the back—and during her tenure, she would add, thankfully, the three more.

In the months after buying the property, calling in someone to plow the snow from the driveway, a plumber, mowers, a pond guy, and the like, after we gave our address and described the place, they would undoubtedly say, "Oh, you live on Yancey's property. I've been there many times. She was quite a character." Almost verbatim. I had been fond of calling our new place the "Delamater Homestead," but it was, in fact, "Yancey's property." It became easier to just tell people that we live on Yancey's property. The stone house itself, though, I insisted, was the Delamater House.

Yancey was an extrovert—and, evidently, a deeply committed one. Everyone around here knew her. And everyone had an opinion about her. High-energy. Gutsy. Adventurous. Creative. I am a gardener as she had been, but one who is an introvert. A devout introvert, serious about my work, focused on my plants, deciphering the ingredients of my salads in restaurants while being a voyeur, a people watcher, in those restaurants, always interested not only in what I'm eating but also in what others are eating.

Yancey lived from her heart. I, from my head. She was a gifted artist. I, a doctor and soon-to-be nerdy farmer. Born in Missouri, Yancey had lived in Kansas, Oklahoma, California, Colorado, New York, Africa, and probably other places. I don't know for sure, as we never met her. She was ill and had returned to family in Texas when we had viewed her home and her property, under snow, and signed the closing papers. She died, with family beside her, a few weeks after we moved in.

Yancey had opened Aspen's first school of art. But, as an avid traveler, she would not lay down roots there the same way she did abroad and, eventually, here. She painted the reds and yellows of Colorado landscapes, and the spots and stripes of African wildlife. Her fabulous studio, the second of two large living rooms behind the old stone house, became our bright and sunny living room, and in years to come, my make-do March and April greenhouse for my first few farming seasons.

Within a couple of years, as I built my farm, plumbers, tree guys, and neighbors began to refer to our place as "the little vegetable farm over on Yancey's old property." They used to call it Yancey's property; now, it's Yancey's old property. The property is indeed quite old, and the farm is in fact quite little.

CDBD : HD AND NINE KIDS

Yancey's left-behind paragraph provided very little detail beyond explaining the cornerstone etching on the front porch: "CDBD : HD : IL" (and, underneath the "CDBD : HD," "1828"). The paragraph noted that her house—now our house—the Delamater House, had been built in 1828; it previously had a frame addition on the left; and the paternal lineage of its builders was French ("Delamaters"), not Dutch.

During the cold winter months, I set about getting to know them. Cornelius Du Bois Delamater lived September 10, 1789, to October 3, 1852. Cornelius was a pretty popular name at the time; back then, everyone knew at least one. The Delamater surname, through the years, would have various spellings and misspellings: DeLamater, DeLameter, Delameter, LeMaitre, Le Maistre. It was French, meaning "the master."

Hannah Slaughter (noted elsewhere as Schryter or Sluyter) Delamater lived August 4, 1790, to February 28, 1868. Cornelius was born just six years after the end of the Revolutionary War, which his father had fought in; Hannah just seven. They married in November of 1809, both at the age of 19. They likely made their home in a small frame house on the large Delamater property of Cornelius's father and grandfather until they built the stone house some twenty years after marrying. When the etched cornerstone was laid, Cornelius was thirty-eight or thirty-nine, and Hannah thirty-seven or thirty-eight. They died at the ages of sixty-three and seventy-seven. Cornelius did not live long enough to witness the Civil War, though Hannah lived through it, here on what would later be named Union Center Road.

Hannah gave birth to nine children. Yes, nine. It was not unusual for the times—or even for fairly recent times, as my own Granny gave birth to twelve. During several cold winters, once all of next season's seeds were ordered and awaiting springtime as I was, I would uncover a lot about the Delamater family, including where they went to church: what was then the Church at Klyne Esopus, erected in 1827 as Cornelius and Hannah were building the stone house. The Delamaters' buckboard trip to the towering Dutch church in Kingston—which is a site to see for tourists in the Hudson Valley—would have taken about one and a half hours, and to the Dutch church in New Paltz, well over two. Given such distances, the community, the congregants argued, was deteriorating, slipping into sin. The Delamater family and several others petitioned for, and were granted, the new congregation just over four miles away along the winding road toward the Hudson.

A GARDEN BESIDE THE GARAGE

Despite several visits in the snow before the closing paperwork, and even while unpacking boxes in April with our new land still under snow, I'm not sure that I had really noticed the fenced vegetable garden, about the size of our two-car garage, immediately to the right of that garage. But by May, I had definitely taken notice of it, and it was calling me. It was calling to be planted. It pulled me in, and there I would kneel for countless hours.

About twenty feet by twenty-four feet, this garden beside the garage is a raised bed in its entirety, bounded by three stacked six-by-six timbers all the way around, giving a depth of over a foot of rich soil—nice, nutritious soil that was yearning to grow vegetables for us. In mid-May of that first year here, after a trip to a local nursery, I easily planted the garden within a few hours. I thought about Granny and her garden the whole time. In fact, just beside the garden sits a large, heavy, rusted iron kettle, a planter now, that had traveled with me from Virginia to Georgia, to Washington, and to New York; a kettle that Granny had used many years ago in making apple butter. Outside, over a fire. With her own apples. Little ugly apples, not the big ones—red and shiny—found in the grocery store. So Granny is always with me in my garden. Now, each year I plant in the kettle the farm customers' favorite cherry tomato variety from last year—something for me to snack on while I'm weeding the garden beside the garage.

In my newly discovered two-car-garage-sized garden, I planted two four packs of green cabbage, about a dozen onion slips, a very short row of Blue Lake bush green beans, a short row of beets, a four pack of romaine lettuce, which I was perhaps most excited about, a short row of carrots, a four pack of yellow squash, a four pack of zucchini, and one Better Boy tomato plant. I had no idea at the time that I had just planted vegetables across eight different families of plants.

Would I be able to nurture these little plants into luscious produce for our weekend dinners? And could I accomplish it only on Saturdays and Sundays, given my demanding Monday-to-Friday work in the Big Apple? Only time, Mother Nature, and my hopefully persisting green thumbs from Granny would tell. I could recall enough from childhood to know that the beans, carrots, and beets would need to be direct sown from seed, that the squash would be happiest if planted into a slightly raised mound, and that the tomato plant would need a cage. Thankfully, there were plenty of old bent-up ones—indicating that they had been heavily used by heavy tomato plants—in the garage right beside the garden. I was not confident that these green thumbs would still work after all these years in classrooms and clinics, despite having succeeded with the celery on the rooftop in DC. I was hopeful but not overly emotionally invested; since it had called me, I figured it was worth a try.

CRYING OVER CABBAGE. A GROWN-ASS MAN, CRYING. TWICE. OVER CABBAGE.

The two-car garage had been built in 1987, two years before I graduated high school, by the home's then-owner of the surname Augustine. And like me so many years since, it's still in pretty good shape. In that first spring here in the Hudson Valley, I had planted the plant starts and sown the seeds in mid-May, and within a month, the garden was completely over run with beautiful plants. It became quite a jungle, with the spaghetti squash, mislabeled as crookneck summer squash, climbing all over the fence and the row of green beans alike. I knew I was growing a plant different from the one I set out to grow, as I knew that yellow summer squash plants are bushy, not viny. But the mishap made us start eating spaghetti squash, and the winter was made warmer with six dinners with this strange new pasta that easily fed us both.

Arriving from the city every Friday evening was magical: all of my vegetable plants seemed twice as big as the late Sunday evening or early Monday morning when I had left it for the work week. The cabbage was beautiful; I was shocked at my ability to grow such perfect heads. Even though I knew that I was doing very little (mostly just some minor weeding, as there wasn't much room for weeds to grow) and that the soil, seeds, sunlight, and rain were doing all the work. I attributed the emerging bounty to my own skills—the green thumbs from Granny had indeed persisted.

Each week the garden elaborated on its shades of green. By late June we were eating homemade Caesar salads with perfect heads of romaine lettuce, and, by early July, grilled zucchini. By August, the spaghetti squash vines had suffocated, one tendril at a time, my short row of Blue Lake green beans. Aside from the beans, though, it was a bountiful summer.

The next spring, I did the same. This season, I switched out the beets for some Swiss chard and shortened the row of carrots to make room for more lettuce. The prior year we had stayed home (in New York City and in the Hudson Valley) all year due to the property purchase; this year, we resumed some summer trips, including one to Europe in early July. We would be away from the house for two weeks for a trip to Italy with eight friends. We asked a neighbor to check in on the house in our absence, and I proudly offered for her to "take any of the vegetables that are ripe," figuring that she would enjoy the yellow squash, the few remaining heads of lettuce, and a handful of carrots.

Upon returning from a fabulous and delicious Italian adventure, I was eager to see the bounty ripening in my garden. Some weeds had become as vigorous as my vegetables, but more alarmingly, all eight of my cabbages were gone! They had evidently appeared sufficiently ripe, and this thief of a neighbor checking in on the house evidently had a taste for sauerkraut. It seemed a silly loss, but when I returned to the house to tell Ken, I had tears in my eyes.

"It's all gone! The cabbage. It's all gone! She took all of it."

A grown-ass man, crying. Over cabbage. Not just a grown man, but a psychiatrist who is trained to understand human behavior and human emotions. I could understand her behavior—I had told her to help herself to any ripe vegetables, and she did—but I didn't understand where these tears were coming from. And Ken surely didn't either. He likely thought it to be quite strange, perhaps some sort of jet lag-related emotional reactivity. He said there's plenty of cabbage at the grocery store. That only made the pain worse.

In shedding those tears—an emotional response that had also taken me by surprise—I realized, though I should have already known, that I have a very special connection to these plants, to growing them and to then eating them. I didn't want grocery store cabbage. I wanted *my* cabbage.

I made no coleslaw that summer.

By the next spring, it was clear that I needed a bigger garden. This was despite the fact that we were only there on the weekends, the zucchini ripened so quickly that by Friday night they were giant inedible clubs after five days without harvest, and we couldn't even eat all of the produce coming out of the garage-sized garden beside the garage. But with a bigger garden, I could have a long row of green beans, two rows of potatoes, and plenty of space for melons and winter squash.

The logical place for my expanded garden was situated on about an acre of flat lawn positioned just past the pond, beyond a small forest of oaks and maples, just down from a stony ridge. I called Charlie, a few properties down the road, who was well familiar with our land through former owners, including Augustine and Yancey. He had designed and dug the pond for Yancey. I asked him to plow up the sod on a perfect space that I had measured to be forty by sixty feet. Like my father had done when I needed a flower garden for snapdragons and zinnias in elementary school, Charlie turned sod to soil, and I had my new garden, probably three times the size of my childhood flower garden. This plowed-up piece of our yard would be where I would grow vegetables across eight families, even though at that time I still wasn't aware of how these plants organize themselves into those families.

It was a good year. I spent as much time giving away produce as I did weeding. I learned that the pretty white butterflies in springtime create inchworm larvae that can devour all of my Tuscan kale in just one work week, and that mislabeled squash plants from the local nursery aren't so uncommon—I found myself growing giant blue Hubbard squash instead of spaghetti squash, and, boy, was it a sight to see.

I also learned that groundhogs love the Brassicas. It's their absolute favorite family, in fact. And here's where the second episode of crying over cabbage occurred. Rather than just two four packs, this year I planted five. I figured that we could somehow eat twenty heads of cabbage between the weekends in the Hudson Valley and the work weeks in the city. They grew beautifully. Within a month, I was delighted to see the heads beginning to take shape. Then, it happened. It was Friday evening, we had just arrived home from the city, and, before even going into the house, I was off to the two gardens, the one beside the garage and the new one that Charlie had plowed for me down past the pond.

They were gone. All twenty of them, gone. Just twenty solitary cabbage stems remained standing, all young heads and all leaves gone. I immediately knew that it was a groundhog, and I immediately felt tears of loss and frustration welling up in my eyes. Everything else checked out, growing well—the giant rodent had eaten nothing else, just every single cabbage plant. I made the slow, shameful walk back to the house, only for Ken to find me crying. He consoled me, noting that we can easily get cabbage at the Saturday morning farmers market in Kingston. I agreed in an attempt to stop the tears. Secretly, though, and with an upset heart, I didn't want farmers market cabbage. I wanted *my* cabbage.

Building the groundhog fence took me twenty hours one weekend, as I was determined to outsmart these New York woodchucks by burying the wire at least eight inches underground around the entire garden. They never tasted my cabbage again.

3.

Brassicaceae

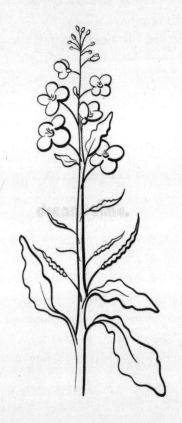

The Brassicas:

Cruciferous Vegetables as the Foundation of Healthy Eating

FOUR PETALS, IN THE SHAPE OF A CROSS, yellow or white. The Brassicaceae family, when left to bloom, proudly displays a multitude of small, cross-shaped flowers (thus also known as the Cruciferae). If the plant flowers and goes to seed, the result is a mass of small bean-like structures with two valves that fall open when dry, releasing tiny seeds. The seeds are indeed tiny, perfectly round, and brown or black. Think mustard seeds, like the kind in old-style, whole-seed mustard. This is the mustard family. This is the cabbage family.

This all-important vegetable family includes cabbage, broccoli, cauliflower, brussels sprouts, kale, collards, mustard greens, Asian greens like bok choy (or pak choi) and tatsoi, napa cabbage, kohlrabi, turnips (and turnip greens), rutabaga, radishes, arugula, and watercress. Tatsoi is sometimes called Asian spinach or mustard spinach because the individual leaves can resemble spinach, but it is definitely in the mustard family and definitely not in the spinach family. Other less-known members of this family include broccoli rabe (rapini), broccolini, land cress (which tastes somewhat like watercress but can be easily grown in soil in the garden), Romanesco, Chinese broccoli, mizuna, daikon radish, horseradish, komatsuna, and wasabi (Japanese horseradish). They are also known as cruciferous vegetables (because of their flowers) and some even as the cole crops (as in coleslaw). This family also provides canola oil and, as noted, the condiment mustard, which is made by grinding mustard seeds (while perhaps leaving some of them whole, for texture) and adding a couple of simple ingredients, like vinegar and salt. It is the healthiest of the three main American condiments.

The Brassicas are superfoods with a great array of shapes and textures. Thus, they are the first of my eight families in my goal of eight on my plate. When counting my veggie intake for the day, I always do so with a goal of eating at least one of the Brassicas. I strive to eat them often and abundantly—perhaps even at breakfast, lunch, and dinner. It's not difficult given the number of family members and their terrific diversity.

Like most veggies, the Brassicas have undergone a long history of artificial selection for shape, taste, growing characteristics, storability, and, in more recent years, disease resistance. Artificial selection refers to humans identifying the most desired traits and then perpetuating those traits in future generations (that is, saving and replanting seeds from some plants but not others). Mother Nature also does this—for other reasons, like pest resistance and general survivability—in which case it's called natural selection. Despite extensive and ongoing artificial selection to optimize the Brassicas, some are more ancient than others. Regular green cabbage, for example, has probably been around since before 1000 BC, whereas Savoy cabbage, again just as an example, is a more recent invention, having been in our gardens and on our tables for just a few hundred years. More on Savoy cabbage later, as it's my preferred for growing and for eating, mostly because it's just so darn pretty.

I really love growing the cool-weather-loving Brassicas in all their shapes and forms. Each plant's multitude of small yellow or white cross-shaped flowers will hopefully never be seen on the farm (that is, unless we are growing them for mustard seeds, canola seeds, or seed saving). The flowers' unfortunate appearance ("bolting") marks their intolerance of any more heat, or said differently, their gratitude that heat has arrived, and their innate desire to push out petals and thus produce seeds. The bolting—flower stalks, then flowers, then seeds—means that our precious produce is ruined since it is the plant itself (roots, stems, leaves, or inflorescence-in-waiting), not its flowers, fruit, or seeds, that we are aiming to eat. Many of the Brassicas have no intention of flowering in their first year. They are biennial plants, meaning that if left in the garden for a second year, they will then send up flowers. Others, however—like mustard greens, Asian greens, radishes, arugula, and mizuna—are eager to flower within weeks of emerging from the soil if sunbeams and the warmth of the soil and air draw the flower stems upward. For those, we must eat them during the cool weeks of early spring, or during the cooling of early fall, before they consider showing us their flowers.

Bolting will again be a concern for some of our other vegetables, rarely for the Alliums, often for spinach within the Chenopods, for all the Aster Greens, and for some of the Umbellifers. We must eat them before they flower. On the farm, planning and timing—and understanding these flowering plants' flowering process—is everything in veggie production.

SUPERFOODS WITH SULFUR COMPOUNDS

The Brassicas contain high amounts of vitamin C, vitamin K, manganese, and soluble and insoluble fiber, as well as glucosinolates, which are sulfur-containing compounds. The ones we eat as greens (like arugula, collards, kale, mustard, and watercress)—or that aren't "greens" but are eaten green (like broccoli and brussels sprouts)—are especially packed with vitamins C and K. The Brassicas are also good sources of vitamins B6 (pyridoxine) and B9 (folate). They provide lots of fiber and are also a good source of protein. Those that are root vegetables (like radishes, rutabagas, and turnips) have a bit more carbohydrate in the form of sugars, though still virtually no fat.

The Brassicas contain some special organic compounds relevant to common folks and presidents alike, as I'll explain. The glucosinolates and their breakdown products, isothiocyanates, are thought to be cancer-preventing compounds. This is our debut of phytonutrients: chemical compounds produced only by plants (in part to help them survive and to keep diseases and pests away) that have health benefits even though they are not required by our bodies in the way that vitamins are. While many are still being studied, a number of phytonutrients are shown by research to be anti-inflammatory, anticarcinogenic, antioxidant, neuroprotective, and immune supporting. With these glucosinolates and isothiocyanates, as well as the fiber and micronutrients, most of the Brassica family can be deemed superfoods. Kale, broccoli, brussels sprouts, and all their siblings and cousins not just are good at promoting your health but also may help you fend off some of the most common and deadly diseases.

The Brassicas are the foremost family of the eight because they are multitudinous, diverse, and very nutritious. They should be foundational to what we eat. But people have either a love or hate relationship with these vegetables. In fact, among all the vegetables grown on my farm, only one has its own list of CSA farm share members who refuse it—a small cadre subscribing to the "No Kale" list because they are unwaveringly convinced that they don't like the taste of kale. Despite ambivalence or outright refusal from CSA members and presidents alike, arugula, kale, broccoli, cabbage, collards, and their siblings and cousins not only are very healthy but can be very delicious when prepared well. The next chapter offers one idea for how to enhance Brassica dishes (spoiler alert: eat your Brassicas with some Alliums).

I like broccoli (when prepared well), so I explored her siblings (like kohlrabi) and cousins (like turnips, especially the cute, petite, sweet, juicy, smooth-skinned ones, like Tokyo Market, Tokyo Silky Sweet, and Hakurei). Since I started growing them, I'm often hungry for many or most of these superfood vegetables, making this first family, regarding my goal of eight on my plate, easy.

Ten or so of the most commonly eaten cruciferous vegetables, despite drastically different appearances, are within a single species (*Brassica oleracea*); they are not distinguished from one another taxonomically, only by cultivar groups. That is, they're not just siblings—they're fraternal twins; and thus have remarkably similar nutritional profiles. Broccoli, brussels sprouts, cabbage, cauliflower, collards, and others are nearly identical genetically, but they take on various shapes. Collards give us large flat leaves; in cabbage, those same leaves are turned inward to form a blanched ball that we slice through; and broccoli and cauliflower are flowering heads, harvested before they send up hundreds of small, yellow, cross-shaped flowers. Because of their similarity, chances are that if you love broccoli, you also love collards and cabbage. Unfortunately, some people despise broccoli as well as collards, cabbage, and kale—it's at least partly a genetic thing.

"'I'M PRESIDENT,' SO NO MORE BROCCOLI!"

So read a headline in the *New York Times* on March 23, 1990. President George H. W. Bush had boldly, publicly declared that he would never eat broccoli again. He announced that he never *ever* wanted to see it, smell it, or taste it again, whether in the White House, on Air Force One, or anywhere else in the country. He had hated it since childhood when his mother had forced him to eat it. And now, as president, he could finally outright refuse to eat it, once and for all.

I'm sure he never submitted to genetic testing, but I bet President Bush was a PTC (phenylthiocarbamide) taster. Probably a supertaster. And had I had the privilege to grow vegetables for him—if he had been one of my CSA farm share members—he undoubtedly would have put himself on the "No Kale" list. Let me explain.

Being a Brassica lover or hater has genetic underpinnings, even though cultural and familial traditions, childhood experiences (like how skillfully, or not, Mom prepared cabbage), and adulthood experiences (like how poorly, too often, restaurants prepare broccoli) are undoubtedly also at play. These plants' isothiocyanates—those health-promoting phytonutrients—are very similar to a lab compound called PTC, which tastes very bitter for about 75 percent of the population but is tasteless for the other 25 percent, depending on the genetics of one's tastebuds. People who can taste PTC are less likely to find cruciferous vegetables— the Brassicas—palatable because they taste too bitter. The tasters can be even further divided into medium tasters and supertasters, the latter finding PTC (and many or all of the super-healthy Brassicas) quite repulsive.

Bitter taste sensitivity is not the same for everyone, and the Brassicas are not just "a little bitter" to all. Central to the story is the TAS2R38 gene, which encodes for the TAS2R38 receptor on the surface of our taste cells—our tastebuds. That receptor is shaped to receive the isothiocyanate compounds in the Brassica plant. Depending on the exact genetic code of your TAS2R38 gene, and thus the configuration of that receptor on your tastebuds, either you can taste the bitter isothiocyanates, or you can't. A minute mutation in one of several spots along the gene (what molecular biologists call a single nucleotide polymorphism, or SNP) affects the receptor's activity such that PTC (and the isothiocyanates in the Brassicas) are tasteless or minimally bitter. Unlike the president, who poked fun at his broccoli aversion on the White House lawn, I am a Brassica lover, and, as expected, I cannot taste PTC when tested in a lab.

Those of us who can't taste PTC and isothiocyanates probably enjoy broccoli, cabbage, kale, and the other Brassicas more than others. To me, arugula is peppery, not bitter; kale is earthy, not bitter; and broccoli just tastes green (if "green" has a taste), not bitter. My genetic mutation allows me to truly savor the Brassicas. I also savor them because I've come to love growing them, and I find good recipes. Plus, my mother and my Granny knew how to cook cabbage—with lots of butter and onions, since bitterness can be masked by fat and sweetness. That's why it's smart to roast rapini and related broccoli-like Brassicas with parmesan and to add honey mustard to mustard greens, and it's why so many coleslaw recipes call for a teaspoon or so of sugar.

Aside from biological differences in bitter taste perception, some people *like* a bitter taste more than others. Do you take your coffee black or with cream and sugar? Bitter sensations are, evolutionarily speaking, meant to be off-putting—a potential defense mechanism keeping us away from various toxic substances that could threaten our health. We are programmed to be repulsed by some bitter tastes so that we don't eat rancid food or poisonous plants and become sick. We'll return to bitter tastes that have made it to the top of Italian cuisine when we arrive at the chicories within the Aster Greens family, like catalogna and radicchio.

A word about adding all this butter and cheese, salt and sugar, and honey and maple syrup to the dishes I describe. I use these supplemental culinary ingredients to make certain vegetables more palatable. But I use them strategically and with moderation. My goal is to eat a lot of vegetables, and if adding flavorings (even those considered unhealthy) helps me achieve that goal, then I think it's a reasonable approach. The key is to not use these added ingredients too often and to not use them so heavily that they turn a healthy dish (like brussels sprouts roasted with a drizzle of maple syrup) into one that's no healthier than a burger (like brussels sprouts drenched in melted cheese, tossed with chunks of bacon, and salted heavily).

MORE THAN AN EIGHTH OF THE FARM

On my farm, Brassicas take up more than an eighth of the growing space—as they should, since they are fundamental to my way of eating and my customers'. The Brassicas are nearly all seeded early in the spring (March 10 to 30), and the young plants are in the ground four to six weeks later. At least that's how I do it in my farm's plant hardiness zone 5b; growing is different in the colder zones 1 to 4 and warmer zones 6 to 13. Most of the Brassicas are ready for harvest within two months. I'm too impatient to grow brussels sprouts (they can take 100 to 120 days from seeding to harvest), and among all my Brassicas, the red cabbage is the latest to mature, at about eighty-five days. The napa cabbage matures much earlier and is usually included in our first or second CSA farm shares of the season; the long green stems of Siberian kale are ready for cutting even before that. Arugula is very quick to grow, about forty days, and radishes are the most expeditious vegetable on the farm, just twenty-eight days. I've come to believe that everyone should grow radishes. Growing vegetables doesn't get any easier.

Among the *Brassica oleracea* (broccoli, cabbage, cauliflower, collards, kale, kohlrabi, and other fraternal twins), the seeds are small, brown or black, perfectly round, and utterly indistinguishable from one sibling to the next. The seedlings are indistinguishable, too, at least for the first month or so, except for purple varieties like red cabbage and scarlet kale. I usually grow four types of cabbage: green, red, Savoy, and napa. The latter, from a different species than the first three (an important realization for both a farmer and a foodie), is probably my favorite to eat. I also love southern-style boiled green cabbage. I've found that kale, kohlrabi, collards, and cabbage are easy to grow; broccoli takes a little more skill; and cauliflower is relatively high maintenance and finicky, with the weather having more of an influence than my two green thumbs.

I love to turn red cabbages into coleslaws or sauerkraut. And napa cabbage makes great kimchi, which is actually very easy to make and stores in the fridge for several weeks.

My favorite way to eat napa, though, is stir-fried in a wok with lots of other vegetables (whatever's ripe on the farm), combined with glass noodles. My preference would be to have it with snow peas or green beans, carrots and/or celery, summer squash, fresh onions, and peppers: six families in one dish! One of my favorite ways to eat Tuscan kale—also called lacinato kale, black kale, or dinosaur kale—is baked kale chips. I should warn you that they can be addictive. Yes, addictive kale, even if you are on the "No Kale" list.

I like growing Brassicas for several reasons. First, even though their seeds are very small—and thus a little tricky when seeding into seventy-two-cell 1020 flats—their germination is very reliable. (The flat sits into a 1020 black plastic tray measuring just over ten inches by just over twenty inches that, in this case, has seventy-two cells: six in the ten-inch direction and twelve in the twenty-inch direction.) Sometimes within a week I'll have seventy seedlings of collards in a seventy-two-cell flat, which equates to a very satisfying 97 percent germination rate. Small-farm farmers calculate germination rates, partly because we tend to be nerds, but partly to help with next year's farm planning. Either the remaining two seeds just didn't have it in them to germinate, or perhaps my eyes (even with reading glasses) were insufficient, and I missed a couple of cells.

I also like growing Brassicas because they are cold tolerant and even cold loving, meaning I can start them early and transplant them out before the last frost. And in mid-October when the first frost usually appears, the fall crop doesn't mind at all. If anything, a frost or two seems to sweeten up kale and collard leaves.

Among the Brassicas, cabbage is my "mother of them all," in part because of its versatility in the kitchen—from homemade fermented cabbage (sauerkraut), to cooked cabbage (stewed, steamed, or sautéed), to old-fashioned coleslaw (best with carrots and red onions; three families in one side dish). While many of the Brassicas are a "one-time-only" sort of vegetable (cutting a head of cabbage or broccoli or pulling out a radish, rutabaga, or turnip), the leafy types can be very generous for weeks or even across the entire season. A spring planting of kale, if kept happy, continues sending out new leaves all the way through October. And the more leaves we harvest, the happier it is. Thus, there's always plenty of kale in the garden and in the kitchen.

The Brassicas offer lots of variety in leafy greens, which is another reason they're the first family on my list of eight. I prefer kale—which we all know to be a superfood—very finely chopped and tossed with fresh, homemade Caesar salad dressing, homemade croutons, shaved Parmesan, and something crunchy (like a diced apple; pepitas, or pumpkin seeds; sunflower seeds; or chopped walnuts).

Arugula is one of my actual addictions. I have a number of them. I especially like arugula salad for breakfast alongside a vegetable quiche. And I like it on pizza for dinner. Sometimes I eat it with just a drizzle of olive oil atop a simple pizza: thin crust, homemade tomato sauce, summer onions, a bit of prosciutto, and shaved Parmesan, with the arugula as the final topping after baking.

My impatience means that I want Brassicas quick. Radishes and arugula help with this, but so does growing Brassica microgreens—eaten as a mix of little two-inch-tall baby broccoli, kale, mustard, and the like. It's an easy way to make any entrée gourmet while also adding a little spice (especially from the baby mustards) and a shot of Brassica super-nutrition. And they're easy to grow in the kitchen.

My biggest dilemma with the entire Brassica family is pests. Compared to some families that have virtually no pests, lots of animals love eating cruciferous vegetables. They must be PTC nontasters. On my farm, which is surrounded by a deer fence, the largest of the cabbage eaters—aside from me—is the woodchuck, or, as we called it growing up, the groundhog. My farm's most dreaded pest, however, is the cabbage butterfly—specifically, its larvae. In midsummer, the cute little white butterflies are flittering all about the gardens. The caterpillar form of this little pest, though, is a green inchworm that eats collard, cabbage, and Tuscan kale leaves faster than I can. And aside from the dreaded cabbage butterfly caterpillar, in the case of radishes, arugula, tatsoi, and a few other Brassicas, the biggest pest is the flea beetle, chewing hundreds of tiny holes in the leaves of a spring crop. This causes no harm to the radish root itself or to the health value of the leafy green Brassicas, but it makes for a less-than-appealing appearance at the farmers markets. So, I grow them under little white tents called row covers.

There is one important unwanted Brassica on my farm: a weed called garlic mustard. I'm not sure why, but some years the garlic mustard seems much worse than others, striking a fear of total invasion. In the first year of its growth, it forms lovely clumps of round, slightly wrinkled leaves. It's easy to identify, but if one is ever unsure, when a leaf is picked and crushed, it smells quite like garlic. It makes a nice pesto. But if the lovely little clumps of garlic mustard remain unchecked (not pulled up by the roots), then in the spring of the next year, in typical biennial Brassica fashion, it flowers, producing thousands of cross-shaped blossoms. And, in typical Brassica fashion, little bean-like fruits form, set to release many seeds in midsummer, blown about and settling into the soil to produce more of those lovely but annoying clumps of weeds next year.

STRANGELY SHAPED AND UNDERAPPRECIATED BRASSICAS

Many of the Brassicas, from arugula to watercress, are underappreciated. And some of them are quite strangely shaped, like Romanesco. One of my favorite Brassicas, being both strangely shaped and outrageously underappreciated, is kohlrabi. Unlike some of the more bitter Brassicas like broccoli rabe and broccolini, kohlrabi is sweet and crunchy. It tastes to me like a cross between cabbage and an apple. I had never eaten or even heard of kohlrabi until I became a vegetable farmer. Even after growing up on a dairy farm with a large vegetable garden, taking biology classes, and going to medical school, I *had never heard of kohlrabi.* That's a serious societal vegetable problem.

Kohlrabi's funny name comes from the German for *cabbage* (kohl) and *turnip* (rabi): cabbage turnip. Its round, swollen stem sort of looks like a turnip, but it sits above the ground rather than in the soil like the white and purple turnip grows. Kohlrabi is much more commonly eaten in Germany and German-speaking countries or in parts of the United States with substantial German ancestry. Although it is a vegetable with a very long history, it was created by artificial selection for lateral meristem growth, which is the "turnip" part of the kohlrabi plant. Like many cruciferous vegetables, kohlrabi is a biennial plant, sending up flowers if left in the garden for a second year—and thus seeds that can be collected. On my vegetable farm, all the Brassicas are grown as annuals; if it were a seed farm, most would be grown as biennials.

Kohlrabi and its siblings were created by artificial selection from the wild cabbage plant, which grows in places like the Canary Islands. As agriculture developed and wild plants were "domesticated," various traits of those plants were selected for, year after year and decade after decade. From an unusually swollen stem just above the ground (kohlrabi), to pretty ruffled leaves that the larvae of cabbage butterflies find harder to navigate (curly kale and Savoy cabbage), to an inflorescence (the full flower head of a plant, from stems to the complete cluster of flowers) with excellent cooking properties if harvested just before blooming (think broccoli, broccoli rabe, and broccolini), these plants have been selectively cultivated over the course of a few thousand years, yielding remarkable differences in looks, culinary qualities, and taste.

ROASTED KOHLRABI, COOKED SAVOY CABBAGE

Given the very large number of vegetables within the Brassica family, I won't describe my preferred way of preparing each when I carry them from the farm to the countertop. But here's my preferred way of eating kohlrabi and Savoy cabbage.

My Roasted Kohlrabi. I usually roast about four kohlrabi. After peeling each one, I slice it into wedges, like steak fries. If it's a small kohlrabi, that might mean four wedges; for a larger one, eight or more. I then toss the wedges with a tablespoon or two of olive oil and lay them out, barely touching, on a flat roasting pan with very short or no walls, like a cookie sheet. I sprinkle the wedges with salt, pepper, and homemade red pepper flakes (or else a very light dusting of cayenne powder), add a heavy dose of shredded Parmesan, or whatever hard cheese is in the fridge, like pecorino, Parmigiano-Reggiano, or Grana Padano. If there's some parsley or chives around, I chop and throw a small handful of either—or, ideally, both—of those on as well, which allows me to count three families (Brassicas, Umbellifers, Alliums) instead of just one. I roast the kohlrabi wedges at 425 to 450 degrees Fahrenheit, tossing a time or two, until tender and approaching golden. It usually takes twenty to thirty minutes.

If you're wondering about homemade red pepper flakes, all you need is a food processor and dried peppers—a variety of your choosing based on how much heat you want. I picked up this happy-making homesteading habit one year when I grew way too many of Jimmy Nardello's sweet Italian frying peppers and poblano peppers. I hung them on long strings in the kitchen for at least four weeks until brittle. Then they went into the food processor for just a few seconds, and out came red pepper flakes (including the seeds), with the dust being chili powder.

Roasted kohlrabi is one of my favorite sides, partly because it is so exquisitely seasonal (early spring and late fall) here on the farm. I roast turnips the same way. The leaves that are usually cut away—from kohlrabi or turnips—can be saved and used along with kale or collards (or mustard greens) in a big batch of cooked mixed greens.

My Cooked Savoy Cabbage. Compared to regular green cabbage, I find that the Savoy's leaves maintain their shape and texture a bit more when cooking. But green or red cabbage is great, too, if that's what I have on hand. I start by slicing the head of cabbage into bite-sized pieces or strips. Then I thinly slice a yellow onion, or, even better, a couple of leeks. I prefer the onion or leeks sliced very thin so that each bite of the slightly bitter Brassica will be accompanied by a sliver of the slightly sweet Allium. Plus, adding an Allium gives me two families instead of just one. I place three or four tablespoons of olive oil into a large, heavy skillet over medium-high heat. Once hot, I add the sliced onion or leek and cook until it is tender and glossy. I reduce to medium-low heat and add the Savoy cabbage, along with three to five tablespoons of water or vegetable stock. I cook it for about twenty to thirty minutes, stirring occasionally, and season with salt and pepper. For an even sweeter dish, I add a chunk of butter about five to ten minutes before the cabbage is done.

I braise collard greens just as I described for cabbage, but I let them cook twice as long, combined with oil, onions, vegetable stock, salt, pepper, and red pepper flakes. Right before serving, I add a tiny drizzle of maple syrup, which balances the slight bitterness of the collards. Or, for the drizzle, for cabbage, collards, kale, and mustard—but especially mustard—I whisk together one part old-style, whole-seed mustard (about a tablespoon) and one part honey and drizzle this sweet honey mustard over the greens. There's nothing like sweet honey mustard on especially bitter mustard greens (of note, the strong taste of mustard greens signals a plethora of health-promoting phytonutrients). And for the Brassicas that are bland (think cauliflower) in comparison to their siblings and cousins, a mustardy sauce can bring them to life.

The Brassicas are the first of our eight families. I've come to cherish spring in part because of my love and passion for growing these diverse cruciferous vegetables. They are super nutritious: superfoods that nourish me and help to keep me healthy. I strive to eat one of the Brassicas daily, or even at two or three meals when possible, and I feel the best about my food choices when I have succeeded. Yes, it sounds extreme, but it's not hard: an arugula side salad (or French breakfast radishes on avocado toast) at breakfast; cauliflower or broccoli with humus at lunch; and cabbage or collards as a side for dinner. With the number of Brassicas available to us, the constellations are infinite. Eight on my plate can easily include at least one Brassica every day—if not more than one daily.

4.
Amaryllidaceae

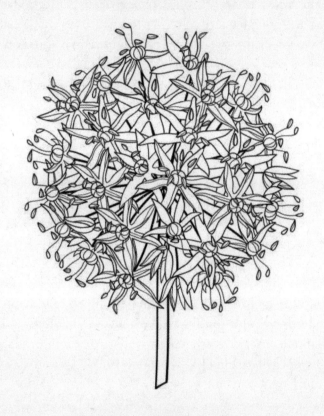

The Alliums:

Ideal Accompaniment for the Other Families

GARLIC, ONIONS, SHALLOTS, LEEKS, SCALLIONS, AND CHIVES. The Amaryllidaceae is a family of plants taking its name from the genus *Amaryllis* and is commonly known as the amaryllis family (as in those large, beautiful flowers adorning so many coffee tables in the winter months). Members of the onion subfamily (*Allioideae*), our focus here, share a characteristic pungent odor produced by allyl sulfide compounds. Sulfur once again. Meet the Alliums.

From a botanical perspective, this family is different from our other seven because, despite being a flowering plant (though I hope to never see most of them flower on the farm, as it means they've gone to seed, thus ruining the root I'm cultivating), all the Allium siblings are monocots, meaning that the seeds contain only one embryonic leaf, or cotyledon. The other seven families have seeds with two cotyledons: dicotyledons, or dicots. This doesn't have much relevance to the culinary or nutritional points to be made, but as a farmer who understands seedlings as well as the finished product, I know that every seed I sow that germinates (and about 80 to 90 percent do) sends up two initial "leaves," though the Alliums send up only one. Allium leaves are linear and blade like rather than broad.

Whereas tiny Cruciferae flowers (on the Brassicas) have four petals in the shape of a cross, the Alliums have a gorgeous, globe-like flower head that consists of a cluster of individual florets (an "inflorescence"), possibly white, but often a beautiful purple. Because I grow onions (and shallots, leeks, and so on) for vegetables and not for seeds, I never get to see these flowers (unless a rogue onion plant sends up a flower stalk for informational purposes), since I don't see them through to the second year of their life cycle.

The chives, however, which are perennial, give us an abundance of beautiful purple globes of edible inflorescences each spring—the only flowering Alliums on the farm. For the garlic chives, or Chinese chives, the flowers are white but equally beautiful.

ONIONY AND GARLICY DELICIOUSNESS

From a culinary perspective, the Alliums are very different vegetables from those in the other seven families because these vegetables are rarely eaten alone. I have favorite ways of eating vegetables from all the other seven families that require few other ingredients—maybe just some olive oil and Parmesan, or a drizzle of honey and seasonings, for roasting. But I never whip up a side of shallots. At the same time, few great dishes lack an Allium, and many of my vegetable dishes begin with one as the sweet first ingredient.

American eaters are very familiar with onions (*Allium cepa*), which we usually classify into yellow, white, and red, as well as garlic (*Allium sativum*). Grocery stores and restaurants have them in abundance because these Alliums have a very long shelf-life once cured, compared to other Alliums, like scallions (which are basically just young onions), chives (*Allium schoenoprasum*), and leeks (*Allium porrum*). If you mainly use garlic and onions in the kitchen, I encourage you to try the related but dainty gourmet shallot and to explore the wonderful leek—my favorite among the Alliums, in part because leeks rarely make me cry.

Onions and their siblings have been used in cooking for thousands of years and across diverse cultures. The Alliums have some, but not substantial, nutritional value in terms of macronutrients and micronutrients. They provide a bit of fiber and protein, as well as some vitamins. Eating the green leaves (as in scallions and chives) provides quite a bit of vitamin K, in keeping with my general rule of thumb that green leaves are always more nutritious than bulbs and roots. For example, with the Brassicas, turnip greens are probably healthier than turnip roots; so, we should not discard the leaves. The Alliums do, however, provide an abundance of health-promoting and disease-fighting phytonutrients: organosulfur compounds like alliin and allicin, flavonoids like quercetin and kaempferol, phenolic acids, and saponins. Such phytonutrients reduce oxidative stress and associated chronic inflammation, thereby decreasing risk for age-related neurodegenerative and cardiovascular diseases, cancer, obesity, and diabetes.

Beyond their own nutritional benefits, the Alliums make other higher-nutrition families even more flavorful and thus more appealing as sides and entrées. They make our other vegetables especially delicious.

GET OUT YOUR GOGGLES

Just as the Brassicas had an interesting sulfur-containing-compound story to tell, so do the Alliums. They contain chemical compounds, produced by drawing sulfur from the soil, that give them their distinctive smell and taste. And those same compounds are why freshly cut onions cause stinging in the eyes, if not uncontrollable tears. The reaction is caused by the release of a volatile liquid—syn-Propanethial S-oxide, as the plant biologists call it—and its aerosol, which stimulates nerves in the eye. It's an organosulfur compound—the S in syn-Propanethial S-oxide stands for sulfur.

Cutting the onion triggers a chain of physiologic events, right there at the countertop and between the countertop and our un-goggled eyes. As the onion cells are cut, they release very onion-specific enzymes that break down very onion-specific compounds, generating, yes, very onion-specific acids. The quick chemical reaction is complex, a sulfenic acid rearranged by a second enzyme, lachrymatory factor synthase, that generates the syn-Propanethial S-oxide. That gas diffuses through the air and comes into contact with our eyes, still, unfortunately, un-goggled. When it does, it stimulates sensory neurons in the eye, causing a stinging, painful sensation. That's the part that hurts. (Of note, some onions cause stinging more than others; for example, sweet Vidalia onions are grown in soil in Georgia with relatively low sulfur content.)

Then, if the stinging pain weren't enough, our tear glands, located above each eyeball—hidden away under the skin between the tops of our eyelashes and the bottom of our eyebrow—take this as an insult. An assault, in fact. They straightaway release tears in an effort to dilute and flush out the sulfur-containing irritant. It's very smart physiology that aims to keep us away from things that might be ocularly dangerous and to help us wash out our sensitive eyes if an exposure occurs.

While the reaction—the initial stinging and then the uncontrollable sobbing—is unpleasant, there's no reason to believe that it's dangerous. The noxious sulfur-containing compounds are nature's way to keep hungry mammals away from Allium bulbs. They keep animals from pulling up, tearing through, and eating Allium bulbs that would otherwise be primed to flower and produce seeds this year or next. Deer, for example, avoid Alliums, and they won't touch the daffodils, also members of the Amaryllidaceae. The tulips, on the other hand, which are from an entirely different family—the Liliaceae, or the lily family—can be completely destroyed by deer while they gingerly step around the daffodils. As noted, the pretty but pesky deer taught me this lesson.

GROWING GARLIC, ONIONS, SHALLOTS, AND LEEKS

At present, I don't routinely grow scallions on the farm, simply because space is always at a premium. But I annually aim to grow plenty of garlic, onions, shallots, and leeks. I also inadvertently grow perennial Allium weeds and one intended perennial Allium, chives. But let's start with garlic.

I plant garlic in late October, or even early to mid-November if I'm running behind, once the soil is beginning to get cold and frosty each night. It's the only crop that I plant in the fall for next year. As a compact farm with limited growing space, I plant each garlic clove (flat part down, pointed part up) close, about three inches apart. The garlic plants begin poking through their winter shroud of straw at the very beginning of spring—a truly joyous sign that life is returning to the farm and to my nearly dormant physiology and subclinically depressed mind. I come close to shedding a tear, no sulfur compounds or lachrymatory factor synthase involved, when I see the rows of garlic arising from the formerly frozen soil in late March.

Growing garlic is magic. It's about turning one clove into one bulb that contains ten to twelve cloves. Growing garlic is about creating a dozen from one. It's magic, and it makes me happy each spring.

But growing garlic is more than just that one magic. Growing garlic is a two-for-one vegetable because it gives us scapes early in the season, appearing in our first CSA farm shares each June 25 or so. A garlic scape—produced by the "hardneck" subspecies of garlic, not by "softneck" garlics—is the flower stalk that grows upward in an endearing, whimsical curlicue, or piggy-tail shape, and that would produce a pretty purple flower if left uncut and allowed to do so. The vernalization (staying in the ground through the winter) cues the plant to want to flower in the spring. But we don't let it flower. We cut the flower stems off, and they are eaten as garlic scapes. On just the right CSA morning in late June, our farm share members receive a little bundle of green piggy tails as a "one week only" special treat. Garlic scapes are why I always grow hardneck varieties of garlic.

Using finely chopped, freshly cut garlic scapes in lieu of garlic cloves is a delight and an indication that the growing season is off to an exquisite culinary start. If you've never had garlic scapes, that's mostly because of this "one week only" issue: they have to be cut, or else the plant will proceed with its innate intent to flower, and the garlic bulb will shrink and become inedible as the plant's energy is expended in the blossoming. Garlic scapes are another good reason to join a CSA: they can't be found in grocery stores, but nearly every small, organic vegetable farm has them—perhaps for one week only.

Here on the farm, the other Alliums are started from seeds, not cloves. Let's consider onions and shallots, which are among my favorite vegetables because, when properly cured and stored, they last all the way through the fall, winter, and spring until the fresh summer onions are ready for pulling on the farm.

My onion and shallot seeds come from onion and shallot plants that have been allowed to bloom on the seed farms, with those seeds then collected and sold to farms like mine, where no such blooming will occur. In seed-production operations, most of the Alliums, like the Brassicas, are biennial (two-season) plants. Bolting (the growth of a scape or flower stem and eventually an inflorescence or flower) occurs in the second year—after a period of cooler temperatures. Here on the farm where produce, not seeds, is our intention, the Alliums, like the Brassicas, are annual (one-season) plants.

Growth of the onion and shallot bulbs occurs when the leaf bases swell to form storage tissue, triggered by increasing day lengths. What I love about growing onions is that there are two opportunities for enjoyment. One is in early and mid-summer when I harvest onions that are in the prime of their growth, with big, bold, sturdy green leaves that are as ripe for recipes as are the brilliant white and red bulbs. These I call fresh onions, or summer onions. They are one of the greatest delights for our farm customers, especially when I bunch together three different varieties, shiny and sparkling. The other type of onion is that harvested in late summer, when the leaves have finished photosynthesizing and flop over, tired and yellowing. That's when I begin a several-week process of curing the bulbs so that they last for months. These I call winter onions or storage onions, like those with no leaves and thin-paper-like outer skins with which we're all familiar in the grocery stores.

Growing onions is all about the leaves. You have to try to relax and ignore what's going on underground while keeping a close eye on the leaves. The more leaves the plant has, the larger the bulb underground will be, each leaf building another layer on the bulb. The size of the bulb soon becomes apparent as the bulb gradually makes its way to the top of the soil; then, alas, there's no more underground mystery. The onions and shallots will eventually sit on top of the soil, just waiting to be gently and easily lifted out.

I grow shallots, which I view as the princess among the Alliums—not just because they're gourmet produce but because they're fun. Magic, once again. They look just like onion plants in infancy and adolescence. Then, the magic starts to happen. Unlike their onion siblings, they form not just one bulb but two, or three, or four, or even five, tightly clustered together. Shallots are durable, too—I often have last year's shallots still in the kitchen when it's time to harvest this year's. Vegetables don't get more generously long-lasting than that—until I get to the winter squash, or—as a segue to the next family—the Fabaceae, or Legumes, which includes the dry beans. The Delamaters undoubtedly stored onions, winter squash, and dry beans through the harsh winters. I've often found myself wondering exactly how they did it, some two hundred years ago, wishing that I could mimic their well-planned approach to the all-important task.

My own cured garlic, onions, and shallots supply me with some much-needed bursts of contentment and pride during long, cold winters. It brings the bounty of the now-frozen-over farm to soups, stews, and roasts of root vegetables and winter squash. I imagine that my curing process looks remarkably similar to that of the Delamaters. The goal is to prepare the harvest in a way that will optimize its storability and reduce rot and spoilage despite retaining juiciness inside. The onions are harvested when the green tops turn yellow and flop over, indicating that photosynthesis and growth are complete. I lay them out in a single layer on a netted structure I designed to fit in the tractor shed. For the next three weeks, the tractor might well get rained on, but the curing onions definitely will not. The key is good ventilation and no direct sunlight. All remaining green tops turn brown, and the skins become dry and papery. A scissor snip to trim the roots and another to cut back the tops to about an inch, and the round onions are ready to be stored in a cool, dry place, again with good air circulation.

I've saved perhaps the best for last: the leeks. Before starting my farm, I never saw much use for leeks in the kitchen. In fact, I'm not sure I even really knew what they were when I saw them in the grocery store. But now, leeks are what I prefer in a summer or fall stir-fry, with a batch of braised Brassicas; with roasted root vegetables; in soups, like the classic hot French *potage aux poireaux* (leek soup), or the similar version that is usually eaten cold, *vichyssoise*; and in quiches or omelets with farm-fresh eggs or egg whites.

For me, the mouth-watering, not eye-watering, leeks are a bit trickier to grow than onions. There's always a portion, maybe 10 percent on my farm, that remain skinny and gnarled and fail to yield the thick, long, white stem underneath a splendid fan of long, flat, blueish-green leaves that I'm striving for. The goal is to get a nice six- to ten-inch white stem, which is the part that's eaten instead of the green leaves.

PERENNIAL ALLIUMS: WEEDS, CHIVES, AND RAMPS

Among the most common and annoying weeds on the farm are the wild garlic and wild onions. They look like a short, slender, clustered Allium plant that, if eaten, would taste like a short, slender, clustered Allium plant, or chives. Just as tasty. Just as healthy. They're weeds because they grow in places where they are not wanted (like in a row of delicate young carrot seedlings), using the soil and nutrients that would preferably be dedicated to other vegetables (like those young carrots).

These wild onions are cool-season perennial weeds that grow from underground bulbs—perennial, meaning they are an annoyance year after year after year. They thrive in nearly any soil conditions and are both cold and drought hardy. Trying to pull them usually results in the stem simply breaking off, leaving behind the bulb (or multiple small bulbs) to regrow. There's no getting rid of them, so I have to assume they are here for a purpose. Who knows, maybe their pungent smell helps keep rabbits away from those young carrots. Like several other weeds in the other families that I'll mention across these chapters (think of the garlic mustard in the Brassica family), these weeds—the wild garlic and wild onions—are perfectly edible, perfectly digestible, and perfectly nutritious. And again, great for pesto.

Chives, a similar perennial allium that is grown purposefully, are always on the farm, positioned exactly where I want and used in lots of recipes, so they are definitely not weeds. They are exceptionally easy to grow, and every home should have a few clumps right outside the kitchen door. I chop them up and throw them on anything, from the garden-variety baked potato to breakfast quiches and dinner pizzas.

There is one wild allium that my farm does not have, unfortunately, even in the woods along the perimeter of the property. I've searched and sleuthed during several early springs, and I have none. I'm referring to ramps. Also known as wild leeks, ramps (*Allium tricoccum*) are a seasonal delicacy celebrated for their pungent flavor and culinary versatility. They're particularly beautiful due to the deep purple or burgundy hues on their lower stems. They grow wild in the woods and boast a unique taste that combines the sharpness of garlic with the subtle sweetness of onion. Although they can be grown on a farm, they are typically thought of as foraged vegetables because of their preference for rich, moist forest soil well shaded by maples, oaks, and the like. I had never been familiar with ramps until I came upon them at the farmers market in Dupont Circle in Washington, DC, in mid- to late April. I discovered that they can be used in various ways to add depth and complexity to dishes (like the other Alliums). They can be sautéed, grilled, incorporated into soups, and used in pasta dishes. Foraged ramps are a prized ingredient in seasonal cooking, eagerly anticipated by food enthusiasts and high-end chefs for their fleeting appearance in springtime markets. Like the Allium Weeds, they cannot be found in grocery stores.

LEEK OMELET, SHALLOT SALAD DRESSING

There's something about the combination of leeks and eggs for breakfast frittatas, quiches, scrambles, or omelets. An omelet and a side salad are great for breakfast, especially when the salad greens are fresh picked and the salad dressing homemade.

My Leek Omelet. I start by thinly slicing two leeks, using only the white and pale green lower portions and not the tough leaves. Depending on the quality of the leek and the farmer's skills and determination, that lower, edible portion might be only four inches, or ideally up to eight. I melt about a tablespoon of butter in a small skillet over low-medium heat. I add the sliced leeks and stir to coat them with butter, then cook them for about ten minutes until they are soft and tender, beginning to caramelize. Meanwhile, I crack three eggs—using only the egg white from one (or from two or all three)—and whisk until they are light and foamy. I add salt, pepper, and freshly chopped herbs—whatever is available at the time, like cilantro, parsley, or thyme. It allows me to count a couple more families beyond just the Allium. I then melt another tablespoon of butter in a ten-inch nonstick skillet over moderate-high heat. Once the butter is melted and coating the skillet, I add the eggs and spread an even layer in the skillet. When the eggs are almost completely set but still a little moist on the surface, I add the cooked leeks and grate on some hard cheese—Parmesan, pecorino, Parmigiano-Reggiano, or Grana Padano. Then, I fold half the omelet over the filling and slide it onto a plate.

Because this is the most unhealthy recipe I'll offer—due to all the butter, cheese, and one or more egg yolks—I prefer to balance the meal by eating the leek omelet with a side salad; again, whatever is at peak of ripeness and freshness— arugula, an heirloom lettuce, or spinach. And I've discovered that homemade salad dressing is the way to go. Store-bought salad dressing can contain hefty amounts of sodium and added sugar, as well as various additives and preservatives.

Making salad dressing at home is quick and easy, providing a fresh alternative that's as unique as each salad. As a chef named Alexa taught me, making delicious salad dressing is about combining six key elements: (1) *oil*, like extra virgin olive oil, avocado oil, grapeseed oil, or walnut oil; (2) *acid*, like red or white wine vinegar, balsamic vinegar, apple cider vinegar, lemon juice, or other citrus juice (the oil and the acid are usually in a three-to-one ratio, though it can also be two-to-one or one-to-one, depending on your tastebuds); (3) an *emulsifier* to help combine the oil and the acid, like Dijon mustard, other types of mustard, or yogurt; (4) *aromatics*, like spices, dried herbs, minced fresh herbs, minced garlic, or minced shallots; (5) just a little *sweet*, like honey, maple syrup, agave, or jam; and (6) just a little *salt*— optional—to further enhance the flavors.

Oil. Acid. Emulsifier. Aromatics. Sweet. Salt. Here's an example of a light, easy salad dressing for any salad at breakfast, lunch, or dinner.

My Shallot Salad Dressing. This salad dressing is so easy to make that I craft it on an as-needed basis so that it is always fresh. Any leftovers can be refrigerated for later. I take a small plastic storage container with a tight lid—or, as Chef Alexa suggested, a small mason jar—and add the following ingredients: about three tablespoons of extra virgin olive oil, about one tablespoon of red wine vinegar, about one tablespoon of Dijon or whole grain mustard, about three tablespoons of grated shallots, about one tablespoon of honey, and a pinch of salt. Shake well until the dressing is well blended. The shallots make it extra delicious.

5.
Fabaceae

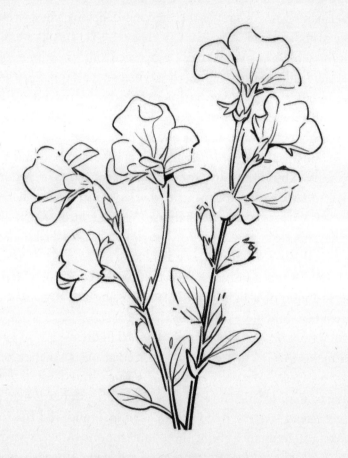

The Legumes:
The Protein's in the Beans

NOW ON TO DELICIOUS, NUTRITIOUS BEANS AND PEAS. And farting and green manure. This is the fabulous Fabaceae family, also called the Leguminosae, which I'll simply call the Legumes. These plants provide key nutrition for us *and* for the soil in which we grow the other seven vegetable families. The other vegetables give us plenty of carbohydrates, fiber, vitamins, and minerals, but here we add a major power punch of protein. This family can give us nearly all the protein we need to happily embrace a health-promoting, plant-predominant eating pattern.

A word about the Legumes' flowers. Unlike the Brassicas and most Alliums—which I hope to never see flowering on the farm—I am delighted for all of the Legumes to flower. That's because, rather than eating the plants per se, we eat the Legumes' seeds or the entire seed pods. Compared to the gorgeous globes of Allium flowers, the pretty, lacy, flat umbrella flowers of the Umbellifers, or the inviting giant orange flowers of the Cucurbits, the Legumes' flowers are relatively unremarkable and often hidden away behind leaves. I rarely pay much attention to their flowers, though I track the growth of the fruit that emerges (the seed pods) daily, waiting for the ideal day to harvest.

A few of the Legumes we eat green—as vegetables; as entire seed pods, like green beans, snow peas, and sugar snap peas; or as fresh, green seeds, like English shelling peas, fava beans, and edamame. But most we eat as "pulses," or just the seeds in those pods, once dried, like adzuki beans, black beans, black-eyed peas, cannellini beans, chickpeas, cranberry beans, great northern beans, kidney beans, lima beans, lentils, navy beans, pigeon peas, pinto beans, small red beans, small white beans, split peas, and many others.

Reportedly, the Neanderthals ate seed pods and seeds from the Legumes, and they've been a staple food across multiple cultures for thousands of years.

On the farm, compared to some of the other families, the Legumes are easy to grow and very low maintenance, in part because the seeds are sown directly into the soil. It's as simple as opening a bag of pinto beans and dropping them one by one into a long, shallow row in the soil, each bean placed about five inches apart. Within a few days, with soil at the right temperature and with the right amount of rain or watering, their two large embryonic "leaves" pop through the soil, and the plants embark on their growing at a relatively fast pace. I only grow a few of the Legumes, given my tight space, but I am grateful to the large farms that produce so many varieties of pulses that I can enjoy in the dining room of this old stone house and that so tremendously benefit my health.

Here, I'll set aside any mention of soybeans—I assume that entire volumes have been written on them—though I'll take a tangent on soybeans when I discuss the various classifications of seeds in the Umbellifers' chapter, since, nowadays, nearly all soybean seeds are GMO, meaning unnatural. But I don't want to talk about that here given my excitement about the other Legumes.

I'll also set aside the Legume we call peanuts—which are not, botanically, nuts—that grow underground in a strange twist of plant physiology called geocarpy. As a vegetable farmer, I know nothing about peanuts, other than that they are strange (though delicious and nutritious). I'll focus mainly on dry beans and, a bit later, on green beans and green peas, the latter including one of my addictions.

PROTEIN, PROTEIN, PROTEIN

Everyone nowadays is thinking about protein, even though the Delamaters had never heard of it, and lacking knowledge about protein had no impact on their way of eating or their health. Here's how I think about it, using veggie smarts, so that I never have to think about protein again. My body makes many, many thousands of different proteins—probably nearly twenty thousand, to be more precise—that carry out my physiological and psychological functions. I make protein. That's mainly what I do. I'm a human protein machine. My different organs make the different proteins needed for their specific functions—like gamma-aminobutyric acid type A receptor subunit delta in my brain, cytochrome P450 family 1 subfamily A member 2 in my liver, and Dickkopf-like (I don't know why it's called that) acrosomal protein 1 in my testes, to name just three among those many, many thousands. To make all these proteins, my body assembles together one or more long strings of amino acids, the blueprints provided by my DNA. That's what a protein is: a long string of amino acids twisted into all sorts of crazy 3D shapes.

Of the twenty amino acid "building blocks" that I use to make all my needed proteins, my body—and yours—can make eleven from scratch. The other nine need to be supplied through food. A few examples of these nine "essential" amino acids are leucine, phenylalanine, threonine, and tryptophan, all of which, by the way, are found in kale, spinach, and other leafy green vegetables.

Eating food that is very high in protein (think muscle, like pecs on pigs and glutes on cows) is one way of getting those nine amino acids. But another way is to eat a diverse array of vegetables, grains, seeds, and nuts, each of which individually might appear to be relatively low in protein (compared to animal muscles) but that together provide all nine essential (dietary) amino acids that I need to make my nearly twenty thousand different proteins, from brain to balls to toenails.

I can get all my essential amino acids without eating beef, chicken, pork, and the like, all of which are both high in unhealthy saturated fat and very bad for the environment when produced in CAFOs that feed the animals GMOs. CAFOs are concentrated animal feeding operations, or agricultural meat, dairy, or egg facilities in which large numbers of animals (such as 1,000 or more meat cows or 125,000 or more chickens) are kept and fed in a confined area rather than allowed to graze, or eat, in pastures, in fields, or on range lands. This brings about challenges related to animal waste, local water quality, and animal welfare practices. I can instead eat things like the following, which, like meat, are complete proteins giving me everything I need: amaranth or quinoa; soybean products like edamame and tofu; Ezekiel bread (made from sprouted whole grains and legumes); and some foods in combination, such as beans with rice, hummus and pita, and peanut butter on whole grain bread. I prefer organic, single-ingredient peanut butter.

PACKED WITH PROTEIN. AND FIBER. AND IRON.

All that said, I still need to prove to myself, and perhaps to you, that these beans give me enough protein. Beans contain about 20 to 25 percent protein by weight, much higher than the protein content of other vegetables. That's a lot of protein. Let's put it into perspective.

Using the USDA's online calculator, at the time of this writing—when I weigh 154 pounds, with a height of five feet and seven inches, at age fifty-two, and deeming myself to be "very active" with free weights at the gym, leisurely biking every day after work, and, of course, daily gardening and farming—I need an average daily intake of fifty-six grams of protein.

So, fifty-six grams. Although I prefer a vegetable-packed quiche with an arugula side salad for breakfast, today it was two poached eggs (that's twelve grams of protein, about six in each egg, though there's nearly as much fat in each of those eggs, a substantial portion being saturated fat), alongside leftover pinto beans (eight grams in about a half cup) and a piece of multigrain toast (three grams) with a big smear of peanut butter (seven grams) and homemade red currant jam. It's a delicious breakfast—and already thirty grams of protein to start my day before the gym.

Today's lunch in the office included some lentil soup, which gives me nine grams of protein. I had a handful of nuts in the afternoon, which is another five grams. Tonight's dinner started with some hard cheese (seven grams) and edamame (five grams worth), followed by a spinach and watercress salad (about three grams of protein) and a medley of roasted root vegetables (probably about two grams).

I've taken in sixty-one grams of protein, not to mention the additional amounts here and there in the other vegetables (like the Brassicas), rice, or pasta that might have been part of my lunch or dinner. It's probably closer to seventy grams of protein. I've clearly exceeded my "recommended dietary allowance" of fifty-six grams, even as someone who is very active—taking hikes, building bean trellises, pumping iron, and lifting bushels of winter squash at harvest time. And I did it without even thinking about beef, pork, or chicken. The Legumes, including those pinto beans, peanut butter, lentil soup, and edamame, gave me what I need.

Many people are overly concerned about getting enough protein, and, unfortunately, protein has become conflated with meat. When the wait staff kindly asks about adding "protein" to the spinach salad, they're probably not referring to chickpeas. There's enough protein in a whole-foods, plant-predominant eating pattern to support our nutritional needs, including our protein needs. I no longer worry about protein.

Beans are also full of fiber. When thinking about "fiber," many think of breakfast cereals and the like, and the grains are indeed a decent source of cancer-preventing fiber. But not as much as the vegetables. And the beans and peas are at the top of the list. A half cup of cooked navy beans provides 9.6 grams of fiber at 128 calories. Compare that to three-quarters of a cup of ready-to-eat bran flakes cereal, which gives 5.5 grams of fiber (at ninety-eight calories), or a half cup of oat bran, which gives 2.9 grams of fiber (at forty-four calories). These beans give us a lot of fiber. I'm not worried about the calories here because they're mostly coming from the high protein content of the beans. All our Legume family members—small white beans, lima beans, green peas, lentils, pintos, black beans, chickpeas, and the like—do a way better job of giving us fiber than do oat bran and most other breakfast foods. I rarely eat cereal, but beans are almost always on my breakfast plate.

Countless other vegetables are exceptionally good sources of fiber, though the fabulous Fabaceae clearly dominate. And we need the Legumes, the Brassicas, the other families, and the grains to give us all our fiber. That's because dairy products contain no fiber, eggs are devoid of it, and meats have none. Zero. Zilch. Pushing any vegetables off our breakfast, lunch, or dinner plate to make room for dairy, eggs, or meats of any type means reducing our fiber intake. And probably increasing our risk of colorectal cancer.

Fiber supplements—capsules, gummies, powder, or what have you—seem strange to me given that we can get plenty of fiber by just eating vegetables. Plus, a fiber supplement must be encountered by our GI system as very strange, as it is accustomed to and designed for food. Perhaps some doctors have reasons for recommending or prescribing fiber supplements, but I err on the side of recommending vegetables, and especially the Legumes.

Finally, in addition to protein and fiber, the Legumes are a good source of iron. A half cup of cooked white beans or lentils gives us 3.3 milligrams of iron at about 120 calories. Compare that to three ounces of beef, which gives 2.5 milligrams at 173 calories, or three ounces of lamb, which gives 2.0 milligrams at 158 calories. I'll take the lentil soup instead of the lamb stew to get the iron I need.

I've gone into a lot of detail about nutrition here with the Legumes (and I haven't even mentioned their folate, manganese, and other micronutrients), despite having said that I'm a just a farmer, not a botanist, and just a doctor, not a dietitian. Well, this farmer also said that vegetables have been growing on me (and on my farm), and that, as such, I've come to realize beans and peas are a true staple of a healthy way of eating. I believe they should be eaten, in diversity, at least daily—or, even better, twice daily, if not at every meal. Among the eight families that I count each day toward my goal of eight on my plate, the Legumes (and also the Brassicas, due to their great diversity) are the easiest for me to check off the list. And switching out meats for beans is good not just for my health but for our environment.

THE PLEASURE OF FARTING AND THE TREASURE OF GREEN MANURE

Farming, or gardening, comes with many little miracles— like turning a tiny Brassica seed into a giant head of cabbage, sowing one garlic clove and getting twelve, or creating a strange hybrid squash like the one Mother Nature made for me one year (though I claimed to have made it; I'll tell you about it). There are two miracles for which we should be grateful to the Legumes. One occurs above ground, the other below. First, farting.

As children, even before we memorized that "King Phillip Came Over From Great Spain," many of us learned the playground song that went: "Beans, beans, the musical fruit. The more you eat, the more you toot. The more you toot, the better you feel. So let's have beans with every meal." For me, on the playground—or, more accurately, running around with cousins in the dairy pastures, careful to jump over all the cow patties (brown manure)—our version was: "Beans, beans, good for your heart. The more you eat, the more you fart. The more you fart, the better you feel. So let's eat beans at every meal." That playground song—or dairy pasture song—taught me two things that we should be teaching our children. First, beans are good for your heart. That might be in large part because replacing animal proteins and fats with plant proteins and fats is undoubtedly and assuredly good for your heart. Beans have no saturated fat and no cholesterol. Beef has a lot. Second, the song taught me that we should eat beans at every meal, or at least most.

The farting part made those two principles fun and easy to remember, but it is also just as true. Regarding the evidently hedonic activity of farting—the more we do it, according to the leguminous lyric, the better we feel. The implication is that we should enjoy the pleasure of farting and should be happy to do more of it by eating more beans.

Here's how it works. Beans are high in health-promoting fiber. Once the insoluble fiber makes its way through the stomach and small intestine to the colon, the beneficial bacteria living there—trillions of them, referred to as our "gut microbiome"—ferment the fiber. Yes, fermentation in our colon. The byproduct of that fermentation? Gas: hydrogen, nitrogen, carbon dioxide, and methane. With just a little effort, thanks to our abdominal muscles, it can be released into the atmosphere. It's way too far down the drain to be let go as a burp. Beans also contain complex sugars like raffinose. Again, fermented by colonic bacteria. And again, more gas: hydrogen, nitrogen, carbon dioxide, and methane. That's some pretty cool human physiology: we need those bacteria, and they need us.

Now let's move from farting to manure—green, not brown. And this time, it's a story taking us from the atmosphere to life underground, rather than from the colon to the atmosphere.

The Legumes are good for the garden because they, in effect, create fertilizer in the soil for the next plantings. It's sometimes called green manure. Most Legumes have symbiotic nitrogen-fixing bacteria in nodules on their roots. Specifically, Legume plants can form a mutualistic, codependent association with the *Rhizobia* bacteria inhabiting their roots. Those bacteria have enzymes that take up nitrogen from the atmosphere, and they share the "fixed nitrogen" with their Legume host plant, the beans and the peas. Nitrogen is an important nutrient for plants and animals—us included—as it is essential to building genetic material, amino acids, proteins, and many other important plant and animal compounds.

Most of the Legume's nitrogen is harvested in the seeds. But there is some nitrogen in crop residues, or the actual legume plants, that we don't eat and that are left behind in the field. Those decaying plants increase soil nitrogen content. It's a natural fertilizer. After the beans are harvested, and the Legume plants in the field dry and degrade, all their remaining nitrogen is released back into the soil as fertilizer for next year's Brassicas, Alliums, and the like. Green manure! Many small farms use legume "cover crop" plants like alfalfa, clover, and vetch between vegetable plantings or when beds are not in production. It's done not to pro-

VEGGIE SMARTS

duce edible crops but specifically to improve soil fertility while also suppressing weeds, reducing soil compaction, and decreasing pest and disease pressure.

For these same reasons, the Legumes play a key role in crop rotation, which is when plant families are moved around each year to different growing areas. As with the other vegetable families, I try my best, despite limited growing space, to move the Legumes around so that they can fertilize the soil across the beds. Importantly, crop rotation also interrupts pest and disease cycles, which is especially significant in organic farming, where pesticides are not used.

THE LEGUME VEGETABLES

I don't grow pulses (dry beans and peas) due to space and time limitations—and because I'm perfectly happy with the bags of dry beans in the grocery store (which are, by the way, the most economical way for me and you to get our protein). When I don't have a couple hours to prepare the dry beans, I'm perfectly happy with canned beans. That usually means canned beans during busy summers and dry beans during boring winters. The main potential drawback to canned beans is that they may contain substantial added salt. So, look for "low sodium" or "no salt added" canned beans or rinse them, as the liquids they're stored in are where most of the sodium content resides.

While I don't grow pulses, I do grow green beans and green peas. The green beans (*Phaseolus vulgaris*, with *vulgaris* Latin for "common") here on the farm include the skinny French filet beans that have the distinction of being called *haricots vert*, the standard but delicious stringless green beans that grow on a "bush," and the yellow wax and royal burgundy beans that add color and fun to CSA members' sauté pans. The burgundy ones are particularly fun because, though purple, they turn green upon being cooked. Magic.

The Legumes' seeds are easy and fun to sow because they're so large. Beans prefer to germinate in warm soil, so I don't sow them until June, and then again in July. The peas (*Pisum sativum*), on the other hand, prefer to germinate in cool soil, so I sow them in April (and again as autumn is approaching)—a row on each side of a three-foot-tall, three-month-long trellis that looks much like a fence. The timing is perfect, as I'll get peas in the spring, beans all summer, and peas again in the fall. Peas come in three types: English shelling peas (the little round ones in bags in the freezer aisle in the grocery store), snow peas (the flat ones in Chinese stir-fries, which might well be my very favorite vegetable), and sugar snap peas. I'm addicted to snow peas. I crave them.

In less than a week, the row of young pea plants or bean plants emerge in their long rows, and, with these Fabaceae siblings and cousins, it's as simple as watching them grow. No tending needed, aside from some weeding. Just watch them grow until their pods are the prefect size for harvest. Harvesting bush beans is done bent over or crawling, while peas can be harvested standing upright and walking along the trellis. For the beans, I return to harvest again in about five days; for the peas, in three days. Both provide a generous, continuous yield for several weeks.

I also grow a special Legume treat for the farm's CSA members: pea shoots. Grown in the greenhouse in the same 1020 trays in which I started the Alliums, a couple handfuls of pea seeds become delicious pea shoots, about five inches tall, in under two weeks. There's nothing like a young lettuce salad with a sliced radish and some pea shoots! Three families. Add some cucumber and tomato to make it five.

UNDERAPPRECIATED LEGUMES: ROMANO BEANS AND YARDLONG BEANS

Some green beans don't require bending over because like peas, they, too, grow on a trellis, though on one that is taller and stays up all summer. My favorite green beans are romano beans: large, flat Italian pole beans. They're crisp and have the best green-bean taste. You most likely cannot find them in grocery stores, except perhaps frozen, but some small farms will have them at the farmers markets.

Yardlong beans—also called asparagus beans, Chinese long beans, and snake beans, among other names—are wildly underappreciated as well. I also grow them on a tall trellis. They're round, not flat, and grow to some eighteen inches or so, as opposed to just six to eight. It's quite a spectacle. One of my biggest thrills is being asked emphatically by a perplexed CSA member, across the eight families, "What *is* that?" (or "What is *that*?"). That gratifying question means I'm increasing my customers' veggie diversity. The strange looking yardlong beans come in green or purple and are splendid in texture and taste. They are technically a type of cowpea, in the *Vigna* genus rather than *Phaseolus*. Again, they're totally unavailable in grocery stores, but a small local farm might have them. My approach to either romano beans or yardlong beans is to first sauté minced shallots or thinly sliced leeks in a tablespoon or so of olive oil until soft and fragrant, then add the beans, cut into about one-inch pieces, sautéing them for just a couple of minutes.

Now let's move from green beans to greens with beans.

WHITE BEANS WITH ESCAROLE, LENTILS WITH SWISS CHARD

With so many options among the nutrient-packed dried beans, one could eat a different variety every day of the month. I offer two simple recipes for flavorful pulses that also add in another family or two, or three. First is my version of the Italian classic: white beans with escarole.

My White Beans with Escarole. My beloved escarole! I'll discuss it with the Aster Greens. I start by thinly slicing an onion and finely chopping a small, sweet red pepper with just the mildest punch. In a large pot, I sauté the onion and pepper in about two tablespoons of olive oil until they are tender and fragrant and begin to caramelize; that's how I start many of my simple vegetable recipes. I add the head of escarole, sliced in about one-inch strips, tossing it together with the onions and peppers and cooking it for just a couple of minutes until wilted and tender. Then, I simply add a can of white beans (like small white beans, or, to be truer to Italy, cannellini beans), undrained, because I like the flavor of the juices. They can also be drained and rinsed, especially to reduce the sodium content. I stir and let it simmer for about ten minutes. I add salt and pepper to taste. It's an easy, delicious side for dinner; it gives me four families (Allium, Nightshade, Aster Green, and Legume); and it's a great leftover for breakfast or lunch. When I prefer to take on a little more effort (like in the wintertime), I start with dry white beans rather than canned ones.

The second recipe is very similar. But instead of escarole, I use Swiss chard; and, instead of white beans, lentils. To my tastebuds, it's the perfect combination of earthy Swiss chard and earthy lentils.

My Lentils with Swiss Chard. I start by thinly slicing an onion and dicing a large, juicy tomato or two. In a large pot, I sauté the onion and tomato in about two tablespoons of olive oil until fragrant. I add a large bundle of Swiss chard, leaves sliced in about one-inch strips and stems sliced more finely, tossing it together with the onions and tomatoes and cooking for just a couple of minutes until wilted and tender. Then, I simply add a can of lentils for the fourth family in this recipe. I stir and let it simmer for about ten minutes. I add salt and pepper to taste. When I prefer to take on a little more effort, I start with dry lentils rather than canned ones.

The long-lasting vegetables and legumes—from cabbages to onions to pintos—see us through the high productivity of summer to the hunkering down of winter. My beets, carrots, and butternuts in this old stone house in February look and taste just like those in the brand-new stone house that Cornelius and Hannah had so proudly built.

Since I've mentioned Swiss chard—and now beets—it's time to turn our attention to a superfood family deserving of a daily serving, with a funny name because of the shape of their leaves.

6.

Amaranthaceae

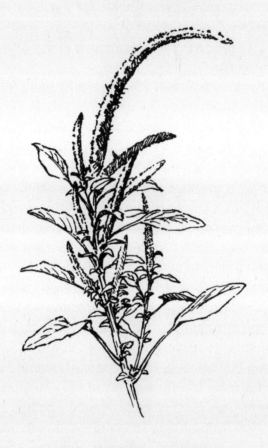

The Chenopods:

The Goosefoot Vegetables as Superfoods

LIKE MANY OF OUR OTHER FAMILIES, the Chenopods—a name that means *goose foot*, describing the triangular shape of their leaves—are a large family that includes flowers, weeds, and vegetables: flowers like amaranth, which is also a vegetable and a grain; many weeds, including some of the most annoying and some of the most nutritious weeds in the vegetable garden; and a few of the very healthiest vegetables—superfoods, in fact. I'm talking about spinach, Swiss chard, beets, beet greens, some nutritious weeds (like lamb's quarters and pigweed), and amaranth and quinoa grain. The family? Chenopodiaceae. And, thus, the surname: the Chenopods.

The family was apparently merged some twenty years ago—as far as I can tell based on my superficial reading of the very complex genetic and phylogenetic research—into the family Amaranthaceae, which has a couple thousand species. On the farm, I grow several species as cut flowers, though they're flowers that have no petals. These include amaranth varieties like love lies bleeding and celosia varieties like flamingo feathers. I really adore those flowers. They add the most endearing character to any bouquet of blooms.

But I'm here to talk about vegetables, not cut flowers, and I'll let other sources give details about the protein-packed, super-nutritious grains (amaranth and quinoa). Among the Chenopod vegetables, we have just three: spinach, Swiss chard, and beets. Plus two power-packed and delicious weeds.

This is hard for me to admit publicly, but I've never been able to grow spinach. I've tried year after year, and it never works. It's an embarrassment. My two green thumbs work for everything else, but the spinach is always a flop. I bet

Cornelius and Hannah had mastered it for both a spring crop and a fall one. I think my failure is driven by several factors: one, my little, diverse farm grows about ninety cultivars across the sixty or so vegetables (not including the fruits and the cut flowers); two, each cultivar requires its own ongoing attention; three, spinach evidently requires a little more attention than average; and four, I have only been giving it average attention. This is despite the fact that spinach is one of the several vegetables that I'm addicted to—along with arugula from the Brassicas, snow peas from the Legumes, fried yellow squash and roasted winter squash from the Cucurbits, and shishito peppers and cherry tomatoes from the Nightshades. I'm seriously addicted to spinach. My condition even meets some of the psychiatric diagnostic criteria for addiction, except that it doesn't impair my life: cravings; finding that once I start using (eating) it, I end up using (eating) more of it than I intended; having a strong desire or urge to use (eat) it (even when out of season); and having withdrawals (necessitating highly disguised grocery store visits) when it is available neither on my farm (always) nor at the farmers markets (in the heat of the summer).

Addictions aside, even though I cannot grow spinach, I can definitely grow Swiss chard and its fraternal twin (in the same species): beets. In fact, Swiss chard is one of my favorite plants on the farm because its stems and leaves are so beautiful, colorful, generous, and rewarding—and exceptionally nutritious. This proclamation might sound strange to some, but here it goes: Swiss chard should be a staple of what we eat, right up there with the Brassicas and dry beans. It is one of the greatest superfoods.

Although their flowers could be considered relatively uninteresting, spinach, Swiss chard, and beet *seeds* are very interesting to me. Each seed can produce several plants. That's because each seed is actually an irregularly shaped little fruit or "nutlet" that contains one or two or three seeds. Thus, each "seed" sown results in the emergence of one or two or three seedlings. Thinning the seedlings after germination results in larger, more uniform roots (for the beets) and stronger and larger plants (for the spinach and Swiss chard).

These superfood vegetables are hardy biennials that can tolerate light frosts and freezes—a helpful trait on a farm in the Hudson Valley. Were they to survive or be kept alive through their second season, they would flower and produce seed. Every year, however, among the hundreds of chard and thousands of beet plants on the farm, only one or two of each typically gets confused or goes rogue by bolting, or sending up a flower stalk, in the plant's first year. I don't mind, though, as it gives me a chance to observe their seed-forming process. For the amaranth and quinoa (both of which can be eaten when young, like spinach), the seeds on the mature annual plant are the part we usually eat.

THREE POWER-PACKED SUPERFOODS, WITH POTASSIUM

Even though the main vegetables among the Chenopods number only three, they are all superfoods, meaning that they are nutritionally power packed. Let's start with the solid-green one that refuses to cede power to my two green thumbs.

Spinach (*Spinacia oleracea*) has high nutritional value, whether fresh, frozen, steamed, quickly boiled, or—as I usually prepare it—sautéed in just two minutes or so. Tons of fiber. Vitamin A. Vitamin C. Vitamin E. Vitamin K. Folate. Calcium. Magnesium. Manganese. Iron. Potassium. And so many other vitamins and minerals, including some phytonutrients that are known antioxidants. Spinach is more nutritious when cooked (like Swiss chard, spinach contains oxalic acid, a compound that blocks absorption of iron and calcium but breaks down under high temperatures), and it loses much of its nutritional value when stored for more than a few days, so getting it freshly cut at a farmers market or CSA is ideal. Fresh is always best.

Swiss chard is *Beta vulgaris*, subspecies *vulgaris*, Flavescens Group. As noted among our green beans (*Phaseolus vulgaris*) in the Legumes, the word *vulgaris* is Latin for "common." Not only is it one of the most uncommonly beautiful plants on the farm, but Swiss chard is one of our greatest superfoods. There's nothing commonplace about it. One of my goals as a CSA operator is to try to get farm share members regularly eating this near-perfect leaf vegetable.

Beets (also *Beta vulgaris*) are the fraternal twins to Swiss chard. The beets we're interested in are those eaten as vegetables, not sugar beets (which, developed in Prussia in the 1700s, contain up to 20 percent sugar content and are cultivated for nearly half the world's sugar production). Beets are especially common in eastern Europe, where they are the main ingredient of, for example, borscht. Beets are packed with folate and manganese. Their earthy taste comes from geosmin, and the red-purple color comes from the betalain pigment betanin.

When buying beets, I always prefer them with leaves attached so that I get two vegetables for the price of one: beet roots and beet greens. Beet greens, which I think of as interchangeable with Swiss chard, are very nutritious. For example, given the concern of the US federal government's *2020–2025 Dietary Guidelines* for our insufficient intake of potassium, the document lists the best vegetable sources of potassium, and at the very top of that list of seventy-eight is a cup of cooked beet greens, which contains 1,309 milligrams of potassium at thirty-nine calories. The beet's fraternal twin, Swiss chard, comes in at fourth place, with a cup of cooked chard providing 969 milligrams of potassium at thirty-five calories. Amaranth leaves are number eight, and spinach is at ninth place, with a cup giving 839 milligrams at forty-one calories.

Back in medical school, I learned that bananas are the ideal source of potassium. In fact, we considered them a "treatment" for low potassium levels among patients in the hospital, a nursing home, or the outpatient clinic. A medium-sized banana provides 451 milligrams of potassium at 112 calories. But our handy *Dietary Guidelines* list gives thirty-nine vegetables that out-perform the banana, spanning from acorn squash to yams, and from artichokes to white beans. Chief among them, as noted, are the Chenopods.

One way to add some raw Chenopod to any entrée is—like I recommended for the Brassicas—to add on some Chenopod microgreens as a gorgeous garnish. Little baby beet plants, amaranth plants, and the like, grown right in the kitchen, add a unique flavor to any plate. Not only are they delicious and nutritious, but they are very gourmet in appearance. It's a guaranteed way to impress dinner guests.

THE POSSIBILITY OF PINK P_ _ AND RED P _ _ P

Now to a warning. Eating beets may cause pink pee or red poop. (Doctors are always thinking and asking about pee and poop.)

This happens when the betanin and related pigments are not broken down by the body and so are excreted. The pink pee is referred to, in medical circles, as *beeturia* (a more sophisticated, Latin term than *beet urine*), a totally benign condition relative to the similar pink pee called *hematuria*, or blood in the urine, which requires urgent medical evaluation.

Beeturia may occur in only about 10 percent of the population the morning after a beet salad at dinner. It can also occur after eating foods colored using beet juice, which is a great food coloring. Beeturia (not concerning) looks just like hematuria (warranting medical attention), sometimes prompting calls to doctors' offices. When dealing with any concern about blood in the urine, we always first ask if there was a beet salad at dinner last night.

I considered here going into a discussion of red poop, perhaps an even more common occurrence the day after a delicious beet salad. But since I've already indicated that the betanin and related pigments can be excreted, enough said. Green manure in chapter five and red poop in chapter six just seemed too much for a respectable book on the vegetables I eat.

CHENOPOD VEGETABLES AND CHENOPOD WEEDS ON THE FARM

Here on my farm, I try to grow spinach, and I fail. It's my only nonsuccess that recurs annually. But I will eventually master it, and when I do, it will be a glorious year. Until then, I will continue glorying in the success of my other Chenopod veggies and my beautiful amaranth cut flowers.

The Swiss chard, unlike the spinach, is always a big success. I grow rainbow chard, each bunch at the farmers market showcasing pink, red, purple, yellow, and white stems. It's beautiful, and I take lots of pictures of it. And then I savor it with lentils. Swiss chard is fun and easy to grow, and it's among the most generous plants on the farm, providing fresh new leaves from the beginning of the season to the end. The more the large outer leaves are harvested, the happier and more eager its inner leaves are to grow, and the more generous the plant will be.

I grow several varieties of beets, including red beets, golden beets, and Chioggia "candy cane" or "candy-striped" beets. Like root vegetables in the other families (the radishes, rutabagas, and turnips of the Brassicas and the carrots and parsnips of the Umbellifers), beet seeds are sown directly into the soil. This makes the process easy, assuming plenty of rain or watering brings about good germination.

As is true of six of the other seven families (all but the Cucurbits, as far as I am aware), the farm also grows

Chenopod weeds. Indeed, one of the farm's most important weeds is pigweed (*Amaranthus retroflexus*), and it is a matter of tradition that we treat it as a weed to be pulled, hoed, and abhorred—unlike its cousin, the Swiss chard, growing right alongside it. I let some of the pigweed grow since it serves as a spinach substitute, sautéed for breakfast or as the Chenopod base of a salad at dinner.

Another Chenopod weed is lamb's quarters (*Chenopodium album* and *Chenopodium berlandieri*). I've known it since seeing it in Granny's garden and ours growing up, so I can spot it from the bottom to the top of a one-hundred-foot bed of vegetables. It's easy to pull up, roots and all. Big farms of soybeans and field corn probably despise it, and, as I'll describe, Roundup Ready GMO seeds are engineered to deal with it. On my little farm, lamb's quarters is the weed of least concern.

As I mentioned, the US federal government's *Dietary Guidelines* call out calcium, potassium, fiber, and vitamin D as potential nutrient concerns for the US population. Given the concern, the *Guidelines* offer examples of food sources to make sure we're getting enough of each of these nutrients. For calcium, as we might expect, dairy products are high on the list, but one of my farm's weeds, lamb's quarters, packs a bigger punch than milk. A cup of cooked lamb's quarters gives me 464 milligrams of calcium at fifty-eight calories, whereas a cup of low fat (1 percent) milk gives me 305 milligrams of calcium at 102 calories. In fact, lamb's quarters is listed by the government as the number two source of calcium, second only to a cup of nonfat plain yogurt, which gives 488 milligrams of calcium at 137 calories. Clearly, we should all be eating lamb's quarters instead of treating it as a weed. It is as delicious as spinach and Swiss chard; it is cultivated and eaten as a vegetable in parts of India, Pakistan, and Nepal. Like pigweed (and spinach, Swiss chard, beets, amaranth, and quinoa), some of the leaves of lamb's quarters are shaped not like a lamb's foot but like a goose's foot.

EATING GOOSEFOOT SUPERFOODS

If you get into a routine of eating spinach, beets and beet greens, and Swiss chard (and perhaps even lamb's quarters and pigweed), you'll come to crave these vegetables. If you grow them yourself, you'll definitely crave them, given your close, loving, caring and nurturing relationship with them.

As you know by now—given my willingness to be utterly frank as a frustrated failure at spinach growing—I must buy my spinach. I prefer to get it at the farmers markets. Sometimes the friendly farmer under the canopy next to ours will trade a bundle of spinach for a bag of arugula. Perfect! I love bartering for vegetables!

But sometimes, especially in the summer when I should be eating my own Swiss chard, or in the winter when I should be eating my own frozen Swiss chard from the summer before, I don dark sunglasses and a low-brimmed hat—as a self-proclaimed but, in this case, quite ashamed vegetable snob—and step inside the grocery store seeking out preferably bundles, but, if need be, bags of spinach. It's not how I like to conduct myself as an otherwise outright unapologetic vegetable snob. But I've got to get the stuff, since I can't seem to grow it myself. What makes it especially ridiculous is that I'm snickering at the wilted Swiss chard as I make my way across the produce section to the bagged spinach.

The beets, beet greens, and Swiss chard in my kitchen, on the other hand, nearly always come from the farm—easy to grow, easy to harvest, and easy to eat. I like my beets roasted: either roasted and cubed on top of an arugula salad, or roasted with other roots like turnips, onions, and carrots (four families in one roasting pan). When dining out in any sort of upscale restaurant, if a beet salad is on the menu, I order it. They are some of the most delicious salads when carefully prepared with the right ingredients, like a bed of fresh arugula with a layer of roasted red beets and some lightly blanched golden beets, topped with some very thinly sliced raw Chioggia beets, a drizzle of balsamic glaze, a chunk of goat cheese, and a sprinkling of sunflower seeds. It's heaven. Or fresh watercress with roasted golden beets, slices of mandarin orange, and pistachios. Or delicious pea shoots with spiced roasted red beets and shaved parmesan, topped with dainty beet microgreens.

There are numerous recipes for preparing underappreciated Swiss chard. But I prefer it with lentils, as I described at the end of the previous chapter. Swiss chard and lentils—as easy and as delicious as escarole and white beans.

SAUTÉED SPINACH, ROASTED BEETS

I eat spinach (and a lot of it, since, as noted, it's one of my drugs of choice) in two simple ways, despite countless available recipes. First, I coarsely chop it for a raw spinach salad. All it takes is a small amount of dressing, a small handful of baby English peas, and maybe a sliced Umbellifer (like celery or fennel) to add a little crunch. Want to add some protein to your dinner salad? A handful of chickpeas is perfect. That's a salad with four families. Add sliced cherry tomatoes to make it six. The second way I prepare spinach is to briefly sauté it. It's very quick and easy, which is important to me because my breakfast includes sautéed spinach (or pigweed when it's young on the farm) at least three or four times a week. The spinach recipe is given below. Lamb's quarters or pigweed can be done exactly the same.

My Sautéed Spinach. In a large nonstick skillet, I drop a heaping pile of minimally chopped spinach (or, if it's "baby spinach," the whole leaves). The pile needs to be large, as it will cook down drastically, like so many other tender leafy greens do. I drizzle the pile of spinach leaves with just enough olive oil to very lightly coat the spinach when tossed (using my hands). I add minced garlic when I'm in the mood for it, providing a second family. I sauté the leaves over medium heat for a couple minutes until fully wilted. It's delicious.

When I'm roasting beets, rather than cooking just enough for a side at tonight's dinner, I like to leave some for leftovers for salads (especially with arugula) during the upcoming few days. So, I make a big batch, using two bunches of beets from the farm or the farmers market, preferably one bunch of red beets and one bunch of golden beets, if both are available. They are both nutrient-rich power foods, though red beets have more of the (red) anthocyanin phytochemicals. The main difference is not in nutritive value but in taste: red beets are earthier while golden beets are sweeter.

My Roasted Beets. I like to make a big batch at a time. I start by preparing my cutting surface and surroundings: the cutting board to protect the countertops, an apron over my comfortable white tee shirt, and the like. Why? The betanin and related pigments add color to all sorts of things, countertops and favorite tops included. I then wash the beets well and trim off the tops (saving the beet greens to add to a batch of lentils with Swiss chard) and cut off the long skinny taproot if it's still intact. Then, I cut the beets in half. I line a shallow roasting pan with aluminum foil, add the halved beets, toss them with a couple of tablespoons of olive oil, and sprinkle them with salt and pepper. I loosely seal the foil and roast at 375 degrees Fahrenheit for about an hour. They're done when a fork easily pierces them. Allow them to cool, and then simply slide the skins off. I eat some immediately and store the rest in the fridge so that I have a supply of roasted beets for sides and salads for several days.

I bet the Delamaters grew and ate a lot of beets, probably a variety known as early blood turnip. It's not a turnip, but it's shaped like one. And, no, that's not blood. It's beet juice. They grew many other vegetables, though not as many varieties as I do here on this same land, since the seed companies were just emerging, and F1 (first generation) hybrid varieties had yet to be promulgated. Preparing and savoring vegetables is so much easier now than in those old days. We should be eating even more vegetables than they did. But we're not.

7.

What My Farm Is About

I HAD TAKEN COUNTLESS CLASSES to become a doctor. Becoming a farmer, on the other hand, was more about vocation, intuition, passion, trusting my relationships with all these plants, and talking to other local farmers. I attended a few conferences to learn from others, and I picked up multiple books on compact farms, no-till farming, permaculture, biodiversity, and the like. And since my farm was organic certified from the beginning (I had built it from scratch and so didn't need to transition a conventional farm to an organic one), I had to study and become highly proficient in all organic requirements with regard to soil, seeds, weeding practices, pest control methods, food safety, and recordkeeping. Planning was key: the exact harvest amounts I would need for each of about ninety vegetable varieties, the exact days on which to seed each variety, plant-out dates, and so on. My whole farm-planning process started, however, with *life* planning.

FINANCIAL PLANNING:
FROM GARDENER TO FARMER

My job in the city was going well. I was growing as an administrator, a researcher, a clinician, and a professor. But Monday mornings were hard—I had to return to our little apartment with a kitchen just barely large enough to fry the squash. By this point, we always returned to the city on Monday mornings rather than Sunday nights so that we would have a third night in the Hudson Valley. This commuting lifestyle was fine in the wintertime but almost unbearable for me in the summertime. During the week, I could just imagine the zucchini growing and achieving the peak of perfection on Wednesday; the groundhog poking his nose—but only his nose—through the fence to smell the delicious collards and kale so frustratingly out of his reach; and the weeds outpacing the carrots.

By this point in our careers, it was important for us to begin planning for retirement someday, and we came upon Beth, a delightful financial planner not far from home. She isn't just a financial planner; she's a financial *life* planner, and thank goodness for that. That evidently means that she helps not just with your money, and saving your money for retirement, but with your life, and living the life you want to live now in addition to the life you're hoping to live once retired. Aside from looking at our current spending (the chief findings being that it's super expensive to have both an apartment in Manhattan and a house in the country, and that we spend an exorbitant amount of money at restaurants in the city), we had to also look at our values, goals, dreams, and daydreams.

Buying a boat for the Hudson appeared high on Ken's list. Building a fruit and vegetable farm was high on mine. I think that both Ken and Beth assumed this meant a slightly enlarged version of my already oversized garden in the flat spot just below the stony ridge past the pond. And maybe that's what my farm is from most other farmers' vantage point: an oversized garden. To me, it meant learning not just about growing heads of cabbage for us to eat (being a gardener) but growing dozens of heads of cabbage, maybe hundreds, along with all the other vegetables, for *others* to eat (being a farmer). We embraced Beth's process. By the beginning of fall that year, we had purchased a lightly used and very fun twenty-six-foot Chaparral bowrider—a great starter boat for Ken. It was a fun way to spend hot, sunny Sunday afternoons on the broad river separating Ulster County from Dutchess County. Around that same time, a local fence builder installed for me an eight-foot-tall deer fence around a three-quarters-acre plot of land, including my new garden, a plot that would now be referred to as "the farm." It was a compact farm—or wildly oversized garden— that would not grow beyond the fence but would grow tremendously inside it.

By the following spring, we had begun planning a move from my job in Manhattan to a position with the state government that would be based in Albany. With that new job, we would live in the countryside full-time. I would be home every night by 6:15 to spend an hour or so in the garden—I mean, on the farm—and I would get to see what a small-scale vegetable farm operation is all about. Despite having grown up on a dairy farm, I had never even visited a vegetable farm. But I knew that I had green thumbs.

AN ORGANIC FARM IN UNDER ONE ACRE

Though I had been gardening since elementary school, my story of farming (growing food for others) begins here on Yancey's property, the Delamater homestead, the Lenape's land.

As I was designing and building the farm from scratch, turning sod to soil—initially with Charlie's plow—the first step toward a farm was the eight-foot-tall deer fence. After the fence came a little tractor and a little greenhouse. I had a friend design the farm's logo, which features—for reasons that should be obvious—a pretty image of a big green head of cabbage.

Farmers are passionate people, proud of their farms, and I am proud of mine. My "vision" for this new little farm promoted "Fresh, local, organic food that is nourishing to the body and to the mind." And its "mission statement" described "clean food, farm-to-table eating, and striving to be a small but delicious part of transforming local food systems so that we can all be healthy and happy with the food we eat." Yes, transforming local food systems. I know it's a lofty goal. But it just means that friends and neighbors are eating produce grown by me rather than trucked in from California. No iceberg lettuce, boring giant bell peppers, green tomatoes magically turned red with ethylene gas, and the like.

The six words that I use to describe the farm—sort of its ethos—are: *Local. Compact. Sustainable. Diversified. Organic. Gourmet.* These are values shared by many small farms.

Local. Obviously, local means that the farm sells fresh-picked, seasonal produce to CSA farm share members and at farmers markets (and, in some years, to a small organic grocery store and a small, fabulous Italian restaurant). Eating food that is local addresses many major problems, like environmental degradation, brought about by the massive industrial food complex. I've heard it said that grocery store produce (whether it's organic or not) travels, on average, 1,500 miles to reach our table. The farther it travels, the less nutritious (and tasty) it is. Eating local allows us to consume food that is in season here at home, at peak ripeness, when it's most nutritious and tastes best. It also supports small farms in our local communities. It's how the Delamater family ate. Local food to them, like me, was grown by them, like me, here on this farm.

Compact. As is clear by now, compact means that I intensively farm in soil that is lovingly cared for. You can't really do that on a giant farm. My farm is small, and my equipment is relatively minimal. The small scale of the farm allows me to do virtually everything by hand. It's laid out in a way that encourages you to walk around the three-quarters of an acre and discover where and how the vegetables and fruits are produced.

Sustainable. Sustainable generally refers to bringing as few "inputs" to the farm as possible—simply said, no chemicals and as little stuff as possible. It also means that we try to produce what we need on the farm. That's where homemade compost comes in, and why last year's sunflower stalks are used in building this year's pea trellises. Sustainable farming also means not creating the carbon (dioxide and monoxide) footprint of trains, planes, and eighteen-wheelers used to move food and supplies. The farm's van rarely travels more than five to ten miles per trip—a good thing in part because I bought it used, quite old, and it might not make it much beyond that. Sustainable means the farm can, theoretically, go on indefinitely and that we'll have virtually no impact on our cherished environment.

Diversified. Being diversified means that I grow as many varieties of fruits and vegetables as I can squeeze into the farm's tight dimensions. Most years, it's about ninety varieties of vegetables (as I'll describe, nine lettuces: green romaine, the freckled one, three butterheads, Merlot, two new varieties each year for trials, and MdQS; and, as I'll describe, the eight peppers: shishitos, pepperoncini, Jimmy Nardello's sweet Italian frying peppers, petit Marseillais, violet sparkle, poblanos, and both a yellow and a red variety of corno di toro). Some years, I also grow a dozen varieties of cut flowers—my snapdragons and zinnias included—as might be expected given my childhood pursuits in my first flower garden. And, more recently, I couldn't resist trying my hand at *Stropharia rugosoannulata*, wine cap "garden giant" mushrooms. Then there are the hens for eggs and the bees for honey. Diversity is built into the very business model for market farms and CSA farms aiming to provide customers and members with *all* their vegetables for the season.

Organic. What does organic really mean? It means a method of growing without chemicals. No synthetic fertilizers. No synthetic herbicides to kill weeds. No synthetic pesticides to kill insects and other animals—the principles of "integrated pest management" are taken to the next level. And, obviously, GMO seeds—engineered to produce plants that can withstand countless applications of plant poisons or that produce their own animal poisons—are not allowed. With organic, we work almost entirely with just five ingredients: soil, seeds, compost, water, and sunshine. Thus, the resulting food is in its most natural and nutritious form. While my produce is mostly drop-dead gorgeous, I warn my CSA members each year that the kale and Swiss chard, for example, might have some holes in the leaves. And that they might find an inchworm in the broccoli or a slug in the napa cabbage. This is simply insect evidence that the farm is organic. Leaves with holes are perfectly nutritious, and ingesting a larva or two never killed anyone in the way that pesticides do. An independent organic certifying agency conducts a yearly in-depth evaluation and inspection to analyze growing practices on behalf of the USDA. The agency comes and looks at the soil, compost, water test results, all amendments like local straw applied, the lumber used to build trellises, seed packets, receipts and invoices, equipment, weeding practices, and so on. The official "USDA Organic" seal is hard-earned, and it categorizes produce in a special class as the healthiest food possible.

Gourmet. Yes, I refer to my produce as gourmet. I made the disclaimer in chapter one: I'm an unapologetic vegetable snob. By gourmet, I mean that I'm proud to bring CSA farm share members and farmers market customers delicacies they simply can't find in grocery stores, like the Brassicas' kohlrabi and mizuna, the Alliums' garlic scapes and delightful "red long of Florence" onions, the Legumes' romano beans and yardlong beans, the Chenopods' beet greens and specialty spinach (not), the Aster Greens' freckled romaine and catalogna, the Umbellifers' celeriac and rainbow carrots, the Cucurbits' Diva and Zephyr, and the Nightshades' green zebras and ground cherries. They're all healthy, delectable ingredients for gourmet meals.

A LOCAL FARM: A FARM FOR LOCALS

Each year, I expand the growing space within the deer fence, and each year, the farm is different. I rotate the families as best I can despite my tight dimensions. I test new varieties. I expand the infrastructure a bit. And I convert more of the flat beds to "permanent" raised beds that will no longer require tilling. The farm has gradually morphed from a backyard hobby to a small-scale but highly productive local farm. It's perhaps the smallest of all market farms in the Hudson Valley, but it's organic certified, growing a reputation, and selling out of our CSA farm shares. Some years have been very different, like when I nerded out on winter squash and dedicated the majority of my growing space to testing fourteen varieties across three species of genus *Cucurbita*. That was the same year I geeked out over the chicories: *Cichorium endivia* (escarole and curly endive) and *Cichorium intybus* (catalogna and radicchio).

My small business farming started during our third year on Yancey's property after we became full-timers at the house rather than weekenders using those two days to escape our hectic careers in the big city. The deer fence was built, the logo designed, the greenhouse raised, and the small John Deere tractor purchased and delivered. I'll call that year "Year One." I mostly grew small quantities of summer squash, winter squash, eggplant, and various peppers, selling a box at a time—for a ten or a twenty—at a local farm stand that specializes more in tree fruit than in vegetables. My veggies brightened their displays, and the payment, as I'm sure they knew, covered not much more than a pitchfork and a couple of hoes for the emerging little farm.

In Year Two, I planted the grapevines (with whom I have a long-term, ambivalent relationship), the brambles (black-berries, red raspberries, and black raspberries, the latter per-haps my favorite plants on the farm), the ribes (gooseberries and white, pink, red, and black currants), and the first half of the blueberry bushes, knowing that all these vines, canes, and bushes would not bear fruit for a couple of years. I built beds, trellises, pathways, and a composting area. I cleared some remaining brush and extended a gravel road. I set out to see if I could provide sufficient produce for sixteen con-secutive Saturdays for five CSA farm share members. That's right—just five. Five neighbors signed up for the venture. That year the gardens were small, and I really got to know many plants and their habits, desires, and upsets. It might have been this year when Swiss chard became what I view as the most important superfood on the farm, and I began typing up Swiss chard recipes for CSA members, lest they feel perplexed by the colorful stuff. I built a pergola for CSA members' pickup; bought a John Deere "Gator" for a quick and fun way to get me from house to farm (and to haul enormous loads of plant material, compost, straw, stones, and more); and had a tractor shed built for the other John Deere. Both pieces of equipment were unnecessary for my tight dimensions. But they were fun.

In Year Three, again with two part-time helpers, the gar-dens expanded, and the CSA grew to nine members—five full-share and four half-share, the latter meaning they could pick eight Saturdays instead of all sixteen (good for the part-time locals who spent half their time in New York City). I also started running around to a couple of local organic grocery stores (and an occasional restaurant) selling boxes of excess produce, like Swiss chard, kale, shishito peppers, and cherry tomatoes.

In Year Four, still losing a lot of money—which I was told by other small farmers is normal for a third or fourth year—I began to focus on increasing production. And by then, I needed a full-time helper from April through October. The farm was still largely a hobby for me—a very expensive hobby. One expense this year was the hoop house. I longed for a long, long hoop house for tomato production (because, as I'll explain, growing tomatoes in the open field is fraught with problems). But I only had room for a twenty-four-by-thirty-six-foot-one, which is what we built: *La Casa dei Pomodori*. It was a lot of work during that wet, muddy April, but by mid-July the structure was full of perfect cherry tomatoes, and the heirloom slicers were right behind them. CSA membership increased to fifteen, and we were ready to start selling at our first farmers market, in Rosendale, just ten to twelve minutes away. Sheri—my seasonal partner in this wild little enterprise, who, thankfully, was a lifelong master gardener and continually gave me advice—oversaw the Sunday market. I preferred to stay back planting, weeding, and watering. We were naïve to the process, but the farmers market worked. And the CSA members were very happy. We earned nearly $16,000 in revenue, though I'm not going to state the expenses, and thus the losses.

Year Five was an unusual year, what with all the masks and social distancing. But the farm continued to grow. By early May, it was clear that we needed a van, and a heavily used white delivery van was what I found. Sheri and I held our first plant sale (which we, fingers crossed, referred to as our "annual" plant sale, as it sounded better than our "first") in mid-May, with signs along the winding road pushing the idea that everyone should be growing their own tomatoes and peppers in this year of pandemic fear. Masked, we sold a lot of plants across two Saturdays and Sundays: eight varieties of tomatoes, basil, fennel, parsley, onion slips, lettuces, cucumbers, squash, melons, peppers, some perennial flowers, and currant bushes. Certified organic! This year, we would be selling at two farmers markets, and the CSA expanded to thirty members (seventeen full-share and thirteen half-share). And this was the year—despite (actually, I think because of) the pandemic—that I started growing flowers, cut flowers both for CSA members who wanted a flower share and for the markets. The flowers were beautiful and will now always be part of the farm. And then, chickens, another stuck-at-home venture to make it through the pandemic. The week-old chicks would grow into hens for homegrown eggs by next spring. This Year Five saw just over $31,000 in revenue. Double the cashflow! And, once again, I'm not going to state the expenses, and thus the losses.

One expense was an indulgence designed to further beautify the beautifully manicured farm gardens and fight the pandemic blues. I commissioned a local steel sculptor to build and erect a giant, colorful steel farmer in the middle of the farm. The statue, standing about fourteen feet tall and weighing something like five hundred pounds, permanently anchored to this land with two four-feet-deep concrete anchors, goes by the name of Victory, or, without preference, Victoria or Victor. Holding a harvest basket in her right hand and the left raised like the Statue of Liberty—but instead victoriously clutching a handful of colorful carrots—my steel farmer signified a much-prayed-for Victory over the pandemic virus; an eventual Victory over food insecurity, which the pandemic had intensified in a way we could no longer ignore; and an eventual Victory over systemic and other forms of racism, which had gripped the country so painfully that same year.

FINANCIAL PLANNING: PUTTING THE FARM ON A BUDGET

After an extraordinarily productive Year Five season, that winter was one of planning—not just the usual planning of seeds with the lettuce porn, but laying out the beds for further improved efficiency. And the careful drafting of a business plan. That's right, the farm was now on a budget. Sam, a Julliard-trained musician with recently discovered green thumbs, would be here full-time for the season, and Sheri would return to run our stand at the Rosendale farmers market. I would continue as a volunteer, at about twenty hours per week, taking no pay. We would grow *more* of what had sold well (garlic, onions, snow peas, lettuce, carrots, all the Cucurbits, and all the Nightshades), and I would force myself to grow *less* of what did not (mizuna, mustard greens, turnips, escarole, frisée, and celeriac). In this Year Six—again with the early May plant sale, now selling at three farmers markets, and now with forty-one Saturday CSA members (twenty full-share, twenty-one half-share and three-quarter-share, and plenty of flower-share add-ons)—the little farm operation achieved its financial goal: from major losses to a tiny profit. We were just over $40,000 in revenues and just under $36,000 in expenses. Now we were in business! Thank goodness for Sam and Sheri. And for my day job.

I won't discuss Year Seven as I wasn't strict with the budget, and the numbers reverted back to Year Five. Once again, losses. Being born with two green thumbs does not mean being born a businessman. But it was clear that an under-an-acre farm can produce $40,000-worth of produce, possibly up to $55,000 with the right planning. That's tons and tons of food. I had discovered that I could feed others.

It was a lot of work, and a lot of learning. The little farm was a huge success from a growing perspective; less so from a business one (though, admittedly, I had not been frugal). My farm met its sustainability goal in terms of minimal inputs and low-carbon-footprint farming practices, but I had not attained sustainability from this other, financial, perspective. I really don't know how small farmers do it for a living. Actually, most of them don't—they do it as a passion, pursuing a calling, grateful for off-the-farm jobs that keep them afloat. We all have a role in helping small farmers achieve both types of sustainability.

CSA SATURDAYS AND FARMERS MARKET SUNDAYS

Growing vegetables for others is very satisfying. I strove to make it look easy for my customers while continuously learning. A big part of that learning meant really getting to know the plants. By Year Three, I had figured out that all the vegetables I grow fall into eight families. It had been obvious all along, since childhood, that onions and chives are Alliums and that all peas and beans are Legumes. But I hadn't known that broccoli and collards and kohlrabi are fraternal twins, cousins to arugula and radishes, or that tomatoes and eggplants are siblings, cousins to peppers.

Brushing up on the basic taxonomy (that stuff about the King being "From Great Spain") of all the vegetables I grow, about ninety varieties across sixty or so vegetables, helped me in growing them. It helped me, too, in eating them. Understanding our vegetables better might be conducive to eating more of them. It surely worked for me—thus my simple premise of eating eight on my plate.

By Year Five of the CSA, I had created a new way of selecting each week's eight vegetables for the farm share members. While most CSAs offer whichever vegetables are at the peak of ripeness, and thus freshness, in that given week—an approach I obviously agree with—I began planning the CSA eight-items-of-the-week around the eight families. I usually chose eight items across six families, sometimes seven, but ideally, across eight different families each week. I was strategic—as a nerdy farmer and as a doctor interested in health promotion and disease prevention—by never giving romaine and radicchio (both in the Aster Greens family) in the same week, or kale and collards, but I didn't shy away from combining romaine and arugula and pea shoots, ingredients across three families that make some amazingly healthy salads. An ideal CSA share would include a head of cabbage (the Brassicas), a bundle of fresh summer onions (the Alliums), a pint of haricot verts skinny green beans (the Legumes), a bundle of Swiss chard (the Chenopods), a gorgeous Chioggia radicchio (the Aster Greens), a big bunch of celery (the Umbellifers), a couple of cucumbers (the Cucurbits), and a pint of this year's mélange of cherry tomatoes (the Nightshades). Eight families, though the CSA members just viewed it as the freshest of produce.

At just sixteen weeks, my farm's CSA season is a bit shorter than most, mainly because I have a very full-time job and anything beyond an eight-month farming season (a four-month CSA) would have led to complete physical exhaustion. Sixteen consecutive weeks of CSA Saturdays and twenty consecutive weeks of farmers market Sundays pushed me and my little plot to the limit. Needing to ensure enough produce not only means a lot of planning ahead; it also means being up even before the chickens are. Since we harvest much of the produce for the CSA on Saturdays before 9:00 a.m. (and before 8:30 a.m. on Sundays for the farmers markets), we have to get to work well before dawn.

RESTING IN A MAPLE FOREST IN LENAPEHOKING

Once the CSA and farmers market season is over—in early to mid-October soon after the first frost has declared a resounding end to the tomatoes, peppers, green beans, and others—rest is much needed. On cold Sundays I would turn my attention back to the Delamaters to learn how they lived, farmed, ate, and ultimately died.

In the early decades of the nineteenth century, life expectancy was very much tied to one's age, unlike today. That is, if one could survive through infancy, childhood, and adolescence and into adulthood, a relatively long life could be expected. If a girl or boy could avoid death by tuberculosis, dysentery/diarrhea, cholera, typhoid fever, pneumonia, diphtheria, scarlet fever, meningitis, and the like (antibiotics were nearly a hundred years away, and life-saving vaccines even further), a family of her or his own was within reach. Modern medicine and public health eventually virtually irradicated those dreaded childhood infectious diseases. Now, modern medicine and public health are struggling with noncommunicable chronic diseases—those caused not by bacteria and viruses but by the way we live and eat.

When Hannah Martha, the ninth child of Hannah and Cornelius, was born in March of 1883—the second of at least nine babies born over the years here in our dining room, where we have served so many friends so many farm-to-table dinners in an era when farm-to-table is trendy and posh, rather than just every night's meal—her own life expectancy, taking into account all those potential childhood infectious diseases, was under forty years. Hannah's, at age forty-two when she gave birth to Hannah Martha, was about seventy years. Hannah Martha lived only to age twenty-seven, dying early, here in the house, most likely from one of those dreaded infections, or in childbirth. Her mother, Hannah, granny to many, lived to seventy-seven.

As I had gotten to know Cornelius and Hannah quite well, through census records, old church documents, and my imagination, I was exhilarated to finally find their final home for these past centuries. They rest side by side in an old family cemetery, hidden away high in a beautiful maple forest just over a mile from the Klyne Esopus Church. His ancient tombstone reads "IN Memory Of CORNELIUS D. B. DELAMATER who died Oct. 3, 1852, Aged 63 years 5 days"; hers, "IN memory of HANNAH relict of Cornelius

D. B. Delamarter, died February 28, 1868, aged 77 yrs 6 mo & 24 d's." *Relict* is an old word for widow. Here, in her final resting place, the engraver had misspelled her married name on her tombstone, one among so many misspellings across the centuries.

I sat for a few minutes, resting on the golden maple leaves between them, wondering what sort of granny Hannah had been. Like my own, she had given life to dozens of kids and grandkids, who had gone on to have kids and grandkids living lives largely dissimilar to their granny's, though undoubtedly often harkening back to her love, partly through the food she made. I bet Hannah had spoiled them with gooseberry pie, like my Granny did me with her fried apple pies. I thought about my dozens of currant bushes, leafless by now, and how Granny is always by my side guiding me on how best to harvest or where to make the prune. Hannah's grandchildren were surely equally connected to their granny through the vegetables they grew, the rows of raspberries they tended together.

Leaving the old cemetery enclosed by stacked stone walls, I felt an even deeper closeness to Cornelius and Hannah, having sat with them. And I had never felt so warm, even as the long, dark winter months were approaching, now that I knew this couple: CDBD : HD.

I had made myself at home in their house as I built a farm on their farmland, all the while knowing that this owned land—theirs and mine—had been home to others. This land started not as land of English, Dutch, or French. It was Lenapehoking.

As I've repeatedly run my hands through the soil, sowing peas, beans, beets, and carrots and planting four-inch-tall kale and Swiss chard and so many dozens of other young vegetables, I've always searched for reminders of the past. Treasures. An exhilarating rusted old nail, a fascinating fragment of brown or green glass, a flat, triangular stone that might be the remnants of a Lenape tool or arrowhead. The initial caretakers of this land, who undoubtedly thought owning land antithetical to their relationship with the earth, were the Lenni Lenape.

8.

What My Farm Is Not About

BUILDING MY FARM WAS A LONG PROCESS. Along the way, I began eating carrots; actually, carrots, celery, fennel, and parsley. I was introduced to kohlrabi. I became addicted to arugula. I discovered leeks, along with the magic of growing garlic and shallots. I learned to grow beans—not just green beans and pintos, but romano beans and yard-long beans. I looked myself in the mirror and faced the man who cannot grow spinach. I came to realize that lettuce is so much more than iceberg, like my beloved MdQS and Merlot heirlooms, and I became nerdily fascinated with radicchio, catalogna, and the other chicories. And I decided against parsnips, simply because they take too long.

The organic-certification recordkeeping and paper-work is tedious but, to me, well worth the effort so that it is very clear to myself and my farm customers what my farm stands for and how the vegetables (and fruits and flowers) are grown.

A FARM WITH NO GMOs

In growing these vegetables, most of my seeds are open-pol-linated (meaning, as I will describe with the lettuces and the carrots, that the plant is pollinated naturally, out in the open, by summer breezes, birds, bugs, and bees), many being heirlooms. But some are F1 hybrid seeds. F1 hybrid seeds and plants are not genetically modified organisms (GMOs). Hybridizing is about combining traits from two genetically different plants within the same species under controlled conditions (by humans) rather than the random conditions in which the breeze and the bees do the cross-pollination. The history of this process of human hybridizing officially began while the Delamaters were in this house—the mid-1860s—with the father of genetics, Gregor Mendel, and his pea plants, though it had been going on long before then outside of the formal science of botany.

GMOs, on the other hand, are created not by cross-pollination but by genetic engineering in a high-tech biochemistry lab. These modifications of the genetic code would not otherwise occur naturally, like the insertion of a gene (from within the same species or from a different species), thus altering the organism genetically once and for all. This has been done in bacteria and in animals (like mice) for the purposes of biological and medical research.

In terms of the vegetables I'm interested in, I have not come across GMO seeds, and the seed catalogs arriving in my mailbox in December and January specifically do not carry them. But then, I don't grow soybeans or field corn.

Although there are a few GMO potato and squash varieties out there, GMOs have had a massive impact not in the world of vegetables but in that of commodity crops (like soybeans, field corn, and cotton). Although GMOs are largely irrelevant when considering the vegetables in our eight families, they are central to so many other foods we eat—like mayonnaise and ketchup, to name just two among many.

According to the FDA, "In 2020, GMO soybeans made up 94% of all soybeans planted" in the United States. "GMO cotton made up 96% of all cotton planted, and 92% of corn planted was GMO corn." Those numbers continue to climb. Nearly everything we eat that is ultra-processed (like anything with high-fructose corn syrup) contains GMO plant material. And nearly all animals used for meat and dairy in the United States eat GMO crops, like field corn products.

Mother Nature didn't evolve these plants properly for large-scale, high-yield, insect-resistant, herbicide-tolerant production, so we had to step in and do it for her. One example? Roundup Ready soybeans.

What's the problem that this genetic engineering needs to solve? Weeds. Weeds grow in the fields alongside the soybeans, reducing yields by some amount. The soybean's genetic code is thus reengineered to allow the plant to withstand the herbicide glyphosate, which is the active ingredient in Bayer's herbicide Roundup. You know—the toxic chemical deemed a probable human carcinogen by the World Health Organization. The one that numerous cities, counties, states, and countries throughout the world have taken steps to either restrict or ban entirely. The one that we spray on nearly every soybean, cotton, and corn plant in the United States. Roundup would usually kill the crop completely (along with all the weeds growing alongside), but the Roundup Ready crops are genetically altered to take it like a champ and thrive.

We can outsmart Mother Nature for a while, but her evolution will eventually catch up. Weeds have recently begun evolving to be resistant to Roundup. We'll need more genes inserted and more herbicides applied. Bayer has Roundup Ready 2 Xtend soybeans, modification that, as I understand from the company's website, allows the crop to be sprayed with XtendiMax herbicide plus Warrant herbicide plus Mauler herbicide plus Roundup PowerMAX herbicide plus Intact Drift Control & Foliar Retention Agent and Deposition Aid for "better herbicide uptake." Corteva Agriscience has Enlist E3 soybeans with three herbicide tolerances (2,4-D choline, glyphosate, and glufosinate) to control this year's weeds and limit the ability of herbicide-resistant weeds to develop. The list goes on. These genetically engineered seeds allow us to repeatedly spray countless tons of herbicides—countless tons—on fields across our country without killing the commodity crop itself. And those tons of herbicides eventually make their way, I would think, into the soil and the groundwater.

There's no convincing evidence that eating GMO-derived foods is unhealthy per se, though I'm not an expert on it. Aside from improving yields, some GMOs are, in fact, designed to make some foods (like rice) healthier. I'm not suggesting that GMO-derived food intake is a danger to health. But high-fructose corn syrup is. And the products from fields repeatedly sprayed with Roundup are. The whole GMO mega-industry exists to allow giant farms to become more profitable and thus to support the ultra-processed food—and especially meat—mega-industries.

(There's also Roundup Ready cotton. That cotton, soon fashioned into our underwear, jeans, socks, and shirts, is sprayed, repeatedly, with Roundup. It makes you want to stop wearing clothes—not necessarily because there's

Roundup on our clothes, but because they're using so much Roundup to make our clothes.)

GMO seeds are obviously irrelevant on my farm, where heirlooms rule.

A FARM WITH NO POOPY FOOD

While it's extremely rewarding to grow so many vegetables for others, the real delight is in eating my own food—a big pile of blistered shishito peppers with margaritas on the back patio, or vegetable lasagna with our own eggplant, zucchini, basil, and tomato sauce, or the spring's first Caesar salad with homemade Caesar dressing and croutons, which is like an early June holiday celebration in our kitchen. The Caesar was especially delicious in 2019 after many winter headlines warned against eating romaine.

"Do Not Eat Romaine Lettuce, Health Officials Warn." This was the strange headline in the *New York Times* on November 20, 2018.

The lettuce porn had not yet arrived (it'll make sense soon), and my 2019 selections of *Lactuca sativa* were not yet finalized. It seemed to be a very strange headline—a very strange thing for health officials to say. I wondered if they had left off a phrase from the brief, five-word warning, like: "…Smothered in Grilled Steak"; "…If It Means Eating Hamburgers"; or "…without Eating Other Vegetables with It."

But they were actually warning against eating romaine lettuce itself. Perhaps they had decided that it is as nutritionally deplete as the iceberg lettuce carried in the same eighteen-wheelers, and that we should eat heirloom lettuces like my beloved MdQS? No, it was not about the nutritional value of the lettuce, nor the food often eaten in conjunction with romaine lettuce. Rather, it was about poop.

The Centers for Disease Control and Prevention had issued a "stern and sweeping advisory," the article reported. "People should not buy or eat romaine lettuce; restaurants should stop serving it; anyone who has it on hand should throw it out and clean the refrigerator immediately." It seemed a very strange warning from the federal agency charged with protecting our health and preventing disease, which, I would think, should be sternly and sweepingly *encouraging* Americans to eat *more* romaine lettuce.

But thirty-two people in eleven states, from California to New York and elsewhere, had fallen sick. The former, of course, is where romaine lettuce is grown; the latter, where it is trucked so that I can have Caesars in December just like in July. The deaths were not from *Lactuca sativa* per se but from a virulent, disease-causing form of *Escherichia coli*. The recommendation was not to wash the lettuce but to wash the refrigerator—after disposing of the lettuce.

As the alarming article noted, *Escherichia coli* "and other pathogens don't spontaneously appear in lettuce fields." That's good to know, as we would need a newfangled pesticide if they did. Or maybe a GMO romaine lettuce could do the job. Rather than spontaneously appearing, the contamination originates from livestock that are raised or fattened up near vegetable farms. The problem was not the lettuce. It was poop. Like cow poop.

The story didn't eliminate my desire to eat romaine lettuce, as it was supposed to do, but, rather, made me want to grow more romaine lettuce. And that's what I did. Green ones, red ones, and freckled ones. There's virtually no risk of *E. coli* on small, organic farms like mine.

A FARM WITH NO DIRTY FOOD

But there's more to dirty food than just poop. The *New York Times* story prompted me to google the dirtiest foods, and lists abound. One ranking of the "dirtiest dozen" has spinach at No. 2—my beloved grocery store spinach. And the Brassicas—kale, collard greens, and mustard greens—are at No. 3. That, after all the fuss I've made about eating more of the Brassicas. One report notes that the vast majority of spinach samples contain pesticide residue, including neurotoxic insecticides that are highly toxic to higher animals, myself being a higher animal. I've got to learn to grow spinach.

Shifting from veggies, let's take blueberries as an example. Glorious, delicious blueberries.

Before I started growing—organic-certified growing—I had never thought much about food potentially being dirty. I had only known of clean vegetables and fruits. But upon attending a fruit and vegetable growers' conference and sitting in on a session on northeast blueberry production—at my first and only fruit and vegetable growers' conference that wasn't one of my usual *organic* ones—I realized that growing blueberries is partly about love and passion but mostly about pesticides. And a lot of them. You need a lot to deal with leaf rollers, thrips, aphids, mites, leafhoppers, spittlebugs, scale, powdery mildew, blight, lygus bugs, blueberry maggots, sawflies, Japanese beetles, weevils, and the like—and, worst of all, the feared and dreaded spotted wing drosophila fruit fly. I don't know what any of those bugs are or if my blueberry bushes are plagued by them. They don't seem to be. But I only have forty-five blueberry bushes, not acres of them, and that makes a big difference. What I learned, at this non-organic fruit and vegetable growers' conference that I should have known better than to attend, is that growing blueberries is all about spraying blueberries. And I assume that all those pesticides pass into the soil and the groundwater before or after the blueberries pass through my mouth.

I sat through the session and picked up a few pointers on lowbush and highbush varieties but didn't take any notes about all the required pesticide regimens, as I knew I would never spray animal-killing poisons onto my blueberries. I was going to eat them, after all, and so were other animals, like my CSA members and farmers market customers.

After that disappointing bluberry-spraying conference session, I went to a panel discussion that I had been much anticipating—on growing melons—at this non-organic fruit and vegetable growers' conference that I should have known better than to attend. They briefly covered new melon cultivars, average Brix (sugar content) measures in recent trials, and details about full-slip harvesting (picking them at the right time so that they taste like melons and not like cucumbers). But most of the session was on diseases. And with diseases, in nonorganic, "conventional" farming—though "conventional" is a really, really poor word choice for non-organic farming—come pesticides. A lot of pesticides. All approved for use on melons.

That particular conference—which was in January, as they usually are, when farmers in the northeast most need social support—was clearly not going to be helpful for my pesticide-free farming, so I spent the next day and a half in my hotel room writing my thoughts on melons and the other Cucurbits. These will be covered in a chapter with no pesticides, in which I will reveal my own risky approach to melon pests: steps one, two, three, and four, the latter acknowledging that the inevitable beetles will arrive, and I will be praying to a higher power that the very gods who inspired the Cucurbit bibles will have mercy. It'll all make sense soon.

I also don't spray herbicides and pesticides because this land is not really my land. Or, at least, I can only very temporarily call it mine. Those farming here after me might well not want me to spray their land. I will farm this land for several years, and then others will hopefully farm it after me.

9.

Asteraceae

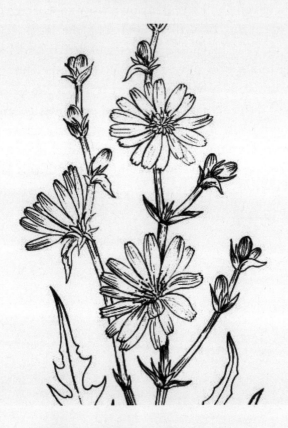

The Aster Greens:

Both Slightly Sweet and Slightly Bitter

THE ASTERACEAE, OR ASTER FAMILY, is a very, very large one, including some twenty to thirty thousand species, mostly herbaceous plants but also some trees, shrubs, and vines, plus many of the most beautiful flowers, asters included. Asteraceae is the largest of our eight families, with the Fabaceae coming in second and the Brassicaceae third. Our main interest here, though—aside from so many of the beautiful flowers grown on the farm (like sunflowers, echinacea, cosmos, and marigolds, not to mention the delightful China asters)—are the lettuces and the chicories. Yes, the chicories. For those interested in the more exotic Asteraceae vegetables, I would recommend artichokes and cardoon, as well as salsify, though I don't cover them here. I like strange vegetables, but all three are a bit too strange for my farm and perhaps even for my palate (but I bet I'll eventually start growing them and then savoring them).

The flowers of these flowering plants are wildly variable. We all know what annual sunflowers look like, and perhaps the perennial purple coneflowers, but what do lettuce flowers look like? Well, even as an avid lettuce grower, I don't know. I try very hard to keep the lettuce from unwanted flowering, and as soon as the heads even threaten to do so (I can tell because the plant's shape starts to turn strange), I pull them out of the soil and throw them into the compost pile. Even a slightly bolted lettuce is bitter, and there's no use keeping them in the ground. I won't say anything further about the flowers of the lettuces.

The seeds, however, from the seed companies, I'm fond of. They're tiny and they remind me of fescue grass seed. But they're even smaller—tiny, but, like the Brassicas, reliable. Germination is good as long as the timing is right, the days still lengthening, and the temperature consistently cool. The lettuces, even more than the chicories, like to germinate in cool soil on cool days. Within two months, I have perfect, large, delicious, loosely packed heads of lettuce, as well as frisée and escarole. The other chicories (catalogna and radicchio) take a little longer.

Although the Asteraceae family is enormous, we'll focus on just three of the many thousands of species in the family. I call these three combined species by their own name (one that I've made up) so that they too have a surname like the Brassicas, the Alliums, the Legumes, the Chenopods, the Umbellifers, the Cucurbits, and the Nightshades. I call them the Aster Greens.

The first of our three Aster Greens species is *Lactuca sativa*. Lettuce, lettuce, and more lettuce! It has been around since the days of the ancient Egyptians, Greeks, and Romans. New varieties were developed in the 1500s, 1600s, 1700s, and so on, with yet new varieties in development to this day. Small farms delight in trying new varieties of lettuce for their taste, their appealing appearance at the farmers market, and, at least in my case, their bolt resistance. That's because I strive to have lettuce available not just in the spring but also, when at all possible, into early summer.

I love *Lactuca sativa*. It is the vegetable that brings me the most excitement in spring, and it's always a huge hit at the farmers markets. The genus name relates to the Latin for *milk*—think lactation (the production of milk), lactose (the sugar that's in milk), lactase (the enzyme that breaks down lactose), and so on. Sometimes when a head of lettuce is cut at its base for harvest, the sliced-through stem exudes a few drops of a sap that looks like milk. Thus, *Lactuca*.

While there are many dozens of species within the *Lactuca* genus, we're only interested in the one, *Lactuca sativa* (*sativa* meaning "cultivated," or intentionally sown and grown, for salads and burgers alike), and not all the various native plants and garden weeds within *Lactuca*. One such weed is *Lactuca serriola*, also called prickly lettuce or milk thistle—a dreaded weed on the farm, mainly because when I hastily pull it without donning gloves, the result is a resounding *ouch*, often followed by one or more—usually more—expletives. Not just prickly but downright painful.

The second of the three species in our Aster Greens is *Cichorium endivia*, which comes in two types: heads of flat leaves and heads of curly leaves. The former is the vegetable escarole (*Cichorium endivia*, variety *latifolia*), and the latter, curly endive (variety *crispum*), is often called frisée. These are not lettuces, but chicories.

In addition to the lettuces (*Lactuca sativa*) and escarole and frisée (*Cichorium endivia*), the third species among our Aster Greens is also from the *Cichorium* genus, this time *Cichorium intybus*. Again, chicories. Here we have a number of varieties of radicchio and the strange delicacy called Belgian endive (or *witloof*, a Dutch word for "white leaf"), and catalogna, which, in the United States, is usually called Italian dandelion. Italian, definitely. Dandelion, not.

So, the Aster Greens family includes lettuce (*Lactuca sativa*) and its cousins: escarole and frisée (*Cichorium endivia*) and radicchio and Italian dandelion (*Cichorium intybus*). As we'll see, in the seed catalogs (porn for the winter months), there are usually only one or two varieties of escarole, one or two of frisée, one or two of catalogna, and two to five of radicchio—but dozens upon dozens of lettuce.

Clearly, lettuce is much more beloved in the United States and has been cultivated, crossed, and selected for extensively.

WHY WE EAT LACTUCA ET CICHORIUM

We eat lettuce because it's delicious and nutritious—but mostly because it's delicious. It's the inverse of the relationship we have with the Brassicas, which some eat because they're nutritious, even if they're not always found to be delicious (depending in part on your taste bud genes). We eat the chicories, also nutritious, for their bitter taste, which is handled magnificently in the right salad and across thousands of years of Italian cuisine.

That's how I characterize the Aster Greens. We eat *Lactuca* because they are delicious and slightly sweet; we eat *Cichorium* because they are delicacies, at least in the United States, and slightly bitter. I'm calling radicchio and catalogna "delicacies" simply because they are delicious yet hard to come by in the grocery store.

Another distinction between the two genera that is also my rule of thumb for the Aster Greens: lettuce never requires a recipe; the chicories always benefit from one. Radicchio recipes, for example, will usually include a fruit like apple or pear, some nuts like walnuts or pistachios, and some amazing cheese like goat cheese. With the right ingredients, the chicories are divine.

These leafy greens, the lettuces and the chicories, are a good source of vitamins K and A. The darker the green, and the more colorful the leaves (pinks and reds and purples), the healthier the plant. The Aster Greens are low in calories, high in fiber, and virtually devoid of fat. Very healthy.

They're definitely worthy of daily consumption for weight maintenance (or weight loss), health promotion, and disease prevention or reversal.

Other leafy greens are deemed superfoods given how packed they are with vitamins, minerals, and beneficial phytonutrients—from arugula to watercress within the Brassicas to spinach, beet greens, and Swiss chard among the Chenopods. The Aster Greens, in my view, are eaten because of their super taste, even if they don't quite top the charts as superfoods.

Thinking about eight on my plate, a salad of lettuce plus frisée plus radicchio, though delicious, makes much less sense from a nutritional perspective than a salad of lettuce plus arugula plus spinach, or frisée plus kale plus pea shoots, or radicchio plus cucumber plus beet microgreens. That's because lettuce, frisée, and radicchio (the first salad), as is now clear, are all from one family, which I have dubbed the Aster Greens, whereas the other three salad options include three families and thus have a much broader nutritional profile. While both the first and the second salad give quite a bit of Vitamin K, Vitamin A, and copper, the second layers in ample amounts of folate and manganese, as well as a broader array of phytonutrients, like carotenoids, flavonoids, and glucosinolates, from the three different families. The third salad is also healthier than the first.

CURLING UP WITH SOME LATE-NIGHT LETTUCE PORN

In my climate zone 5b, in this old stone house in which I do wintertime writing, November through February to me are too cold, too dark, and too dead. I feel bored, restless, a bit numb not just in my toes and fingers, and verging on depressed. It's a subclinical depression, caused by the loss of abundant life on the farm and the cognitive dilemma of the long wait until March, April, and May. I don't always notice myself slipping into the mild depression as each day gets shorter and each night colder in late autumn. It's gradual. It's also both physical (I become pale, have strange cravings for citrus in the absence of currants and tomatoes, feel sluggish, and gain about five pounds despite trying to exercise well at the gym) and mental (as noted, bored, numb, and not necessarily sad but definitely not happy). The nights seem especially long—one only needs so many hours of darkness and so much sleep.

Every year, I only fully realize that I have been subclinically depressed, both physically and mentally, when spring begins to arrive. When the garlic appears from its slumber, I feel myself awakening from a haze I hadn't fully known I was in. When the black raspberries start pushing out buds, I feel bursts of energy returning to my body and my mind, sensations I had forgotten since the same time last year. When the greenhouse is completely full of quickly growing seedlings, I have a rush of renewed motivation and ambition, fully awake, taking part in the push of spring, feeling the renewal of life, wanting only so many hours of sleep because there's so much to do on the farm, taking sick days at work and not disclosing that it's a diagnosable case of spring fever.

During the cold and dark months, on the other hand, as I push myself the best I can to eat well, stay active, and write decently (not using too many dirty words), periodic antidepressants arrive, thank goodness, in the mail. These packages are always much anticipated yet unexpected, spaced apart over a couple of months as if the timing is carefully planned by the companies sending them to keep the small farmers holding onto life until life returns to the farm.

These antidepressants that I'm talking about are, of course, the seed catalogs.

Beautiful pictures of countless varieties of produce across all eight families and a few others. Varieties that I know very well, and new cultivars that were winners in the seed farms' trials last year. They are not technically porn magazines, but there are indeed late-night peeks that do in fact lead to fantasies about growing. All those lettuces! And ooh la la, those splendid new varieties of gorgeous eggplant! The arrival of these seed catalogs is relevant here because it gets to the issue of *Lactuca* equals delicious and *Cichorium* equals delicacy, at least in my farmer-nerd way of thinking.

I receive about six different seed catalogs, arriving as much-needed surprises in the mail on cold, dark evenings when I need them most, usually during December and January. The sexy pictures of luscious, mouth-watering vegetables are ordered roughly alphabetically, starting with artichokes, beans, beets, and broccoli and ending with tomatoes, turnips, watermelon, and winter squash. In some cases, though, the turnips are lumped under a horticultural type ("root vegetables"), and the winter squash might be together with the summer squash in a "squash" section. The vegetables are partly organized around our families (for example, the "Asian greens and mustards" are all varieties of Brassicas), but, in other cases, culinary types trump genus and species (like "Specialty greens," which might include arugula, beet greens, and escarole, none of which are related to one another aside from being flowering plants). Regardless of how the sections are organized, with the sexy porn mag in hand, it's time to officially start planning the vegetable varieties for spring's beds. Farming is about planning—planning while considering Mother Nature's parameters, key among them, in my zone 5b, being the last frost and the first frost. I eagerly anticipate the last, and I always dread the first.

THE SEED CATALOG: THE LONGEST SECTION AND THE SHORTEST SECTION

The lettuce section is usually one of the very longest, right up there with the tomatoes. Delectable mini/gem lettuces, red leaf lettuces, romaine lettuces, and butterheads. My favorite seed catalog, in its most recent edition, had fifty-one varieties of lettuce. That's a lot to choose from, especially for a small farm that usually grows only about nine varieties.

The antidepressant effect kicks in, and I cuddle up by the fireplace with the mag to select my favorite pics, or next year's cultivars. I know that I want one romaine and at least five sweet head lettuces. I review my notes from the prior three or four years: germination rates, how well they held up in the field, how easy they were to harvest, how well they held up at the farmers market, how well they *sold* at the farmers market, and, of course, taste, based on my own taste buds and recorded comments of customers. Each year, the selection is not easy, drawing just nine or so from the more than fifty. I'll want to test new varieties, and I'll find irresistible the heirlooms for which I've developed a fetish, like mouth-watering MdQS (Merveille des Quatre Saisons).

In my favorite seed catalog, forty-eight of the lettuces are deemed OP (open pollinated) and three, also open pollinated, are designated as heirlooms. "Open pollinated" means that the plant is pollinated naturally, out in the open, by summer breezes, birds, bugs, and bees. No human intervention is required. Another characteristic of open pollinated varieties (and the special open pollinated varieties that are deemed to be heirlooms) is that they breed true. This means that—as long as pollen is not shared between different varieties within the same species in your garden—you can collect their seeds and sow those seeds the following year, and they will yield the same characteristics as the parents from which the seed came. Identical. Year after year after year. Many open pollinated varieties are relatively new (in recent decades) and thus not heirlooms (yet). They have been created through artificial selection, resulting in plants exhibiting superior growth habit, heat or cold tolerance, vigor, disease resistance, uniformity, and taste, among other qualities. Many varieties, including many of our lettuces, have been selected for and created in this way in recent decades.

My splayed open seed catalog, the first that happened to arrive this winter, has three open pollinated lettuces that have gained the distinction of being "heirloom": Rouge d'Hiver (red winter), Freckles, and Pirat. Rouge d'Hiver is a French heirloom. Heirloom vegetable varieties are very old ones, grown across many generations—if not centuries— whose seeds are cherished and passed down. From Granny. And from her granny, and from her granny, and so it goes. All the Delamaters' seeds, and vegetables, would have been heirlooms.

Freckles is a green romaine variety that has, as you might have suspected, red freckles. As far as I can tell, it's the same as Forellenschluss lettuce (German for "speckled trout"), an Austrian heirloom. Pirat, a German heirloom, is a butterhead that is, surprisingly, relatively heat tolerant, meaning relatively bolt resistant. It also has beautiful red leaf tips like Rouge d'Hiver. My catalogue explains that Rouge d'Hiver "performs best in the cool weather of fall or winter"—which is code for bolting with any significant heat—and has "red and deep red tips sitting on a dark green base." These heirlooms have outstanding flavor and texture. My preferred heirloom in recent seasons, MdQS, does not appear in this particular catalog, though it's pictured alongside other open pollinated and heirloom varieties in other porn mags.

Horticultural and legal definitions aside, the heirloom designation basically means that the variety has been around for a long time because it is so beloved. All heirlooms are open pollinated, but only a few open pollinated varieties can be considered heirlooms. This is true whether we're talking about lettuce or carrots or cucumbers or eggplants, not to mention tomatoes. Despite their being so delicious, heirloom lettuces are usually not produced commercially and thus are not available at the grocery store, mostly because they are so delicate. It's yet another reason to join a CSA or shop at farmers markets.

So, fifty-one varieties of *Lactuca sativa* for my little farm to choose from, just in the first antidepressant to arrive this winter. And there will be dozens of other varieties featured in the others. I must have a green romaine, as well as the freckled one, and three butterheads. And, like last year, I need Merlot, a giant, loose head lettuce that really is as dark as a glass of Merlot due to its anthocyanin content—a phytonutrient with health-promoting antioxidant properties. I always test at least two that are new to the farm, mainly to understand their growth style, bolt resistance, and taste. As a curious farmer, I get to eat lots of salads, many stripped down to just the lettuce itself with a very light dressing. This helps me decide on next year's cadre of lettuces for my little plot. I've selected eight (plus MdQS), though it hasn't been as easy as I've suggested here—deciding on my lettuces took several hours. As I mentioned, farming is about planning. This farmer, like your own local farmer operating a CSA, has arrived painstakingly at the ideal lettuces for our spring and early summer plates and palates.

Not in the lettuce section, but in most others, some of the seeds are neither open pollinated nor heirloom but are instead labeled F1 (first generation) and/or hybrid. More on F1 hybrid seeds in the next chapter on carrots, celery, and the like (the Umbellifers), and more when I get to the Cucurbits and the Nightshades.

Now I flip back a few pages in the mag to the "Greens, Specialty" section to see the offerings from within our *Cichorium endivia* and *Cichorium intybus* species. Among the endives, we have one variety of escarole and three varieties of frisée. Some seed catalogs don't even have that many. It's a short section since most Americans have yet to embrace the deliciousness of the chicories. And among the *intybus*, we have six varieties of radicchio, as well as one strange addition in this year's catalog, the catalogna variety called puntarelle, a real Italian delicacy. No regular catalogna in this particular catalog, and no radicchio suggested to be grown as Belgian endive. I'll have to find those seeds elsewhere. Surely, another antidepressant will arrive next week, much to my delight, and the planning will be further refined.

THE ASTER GREENS ON MY FARM AND IN MY KITCHEN

My biggest challenge to growing specialty, gourmet lettuce is that it experiences the opposite of my seasonal depressive disorder. Its mood changes, becoming impatient, obstinate, and irritable with too much heat. Unlike me, it actually loves cool temperatures, and, unlike me, it gets frustrated with too much sun and heat. My proclivities for seasons are more aligned with the sun- and heat-loving Cucurbits and Nightshades. But as the days lengthen and become warmer as summer approaches, many *Lactuca* varieties tend to bolt, reshaping themselves in preparation to send up a flower stem that then renders the head of lettuce strange in appearance and bitter in taste, good only for the compost pile. I dare not sell farm customers a head of lettuce that has even begun to think about flowering.

The chicories, except for escarole, are much more tolerant of some heat, rarely bolting, though every year a few of the hundreds of Italian dandelion plants prefer to show us their delightful blue flowers, which are exactly the same as the blue sailors I loved in the cow pastures growing up. Yes, blue sailors in cow pastures. The Delamater kids two hundred years ago here on this homestead would've known exactly what I'm talking about. I'm referring to common chicory, which is the wild version of Italian dandelion.

Aside from the annual bolting concern with late spring and early summer lettuce, I adore the Aster Greens in part because they tend to grow perfectly and without pests. The Brassicas can be plagued by the early summer flea beetles and then the onslaught of mid-summer cabbage butterflies and their inchworm larvae. The Cucurbits, as I'll explain, can be decimated by cucumber beetles, squash mosaic virus, bacterial wilt, and the like. But the Aster Greens—both those slightly sweet (*Lactuca*) and those slightly bitter (*Cichoria*)— always seem to turn out flawless without a bug or beetle or worm to be found. They're so flawless that I have countless photographs of giant heads of perfect lettuces, frisée, radicchio, and the others. I experience a great sense of pride and accomplishment in growing these salad greens. It helps me, annually, move beyond and not belabor my utter failure at growing spinach. Growing lettuce, escarole, and frisée is an easy boost to my self-esteem.

In my kitchen, when I think lettuces, I think delicate leaves and delicate salads—the lightest of dressings, plus a few toppings from several other families that complement the lettuce's sweet and tender taste. Recall the salad I built in chapter one: MdQS, sliced celery, and a sliced French breakfast radish. Once into early summer, if the few remaining MdQS heads have yet to begin thinking about bolting, I might add a sliced Campari tomato and a few cut green beans. That's a salad of five families all built upon the foundation of this sweet, delicate, delectable lettuce. Add a sliced Diva cucumber and I have six families. A third of a cup of chickpeas makes seven. Sprinkle on some sliced scallions and I have eight. Extraordinarily healthy. Food can't get healthier than that.

Some of my favorite lettuce salad toppings, aside from vegetables from other families, include a few shavings of hard cheese, homemade croutons made with whatever bread is available in the kitchen, sunflower seeds, pepitas (pumpkin seeds), chopped walnuts, and a hard-boiled egg. The variations are countless.

To really get to know my lettuce varieties, I sometimes eat them completely naked—simple and plain, perhaps with just the lightest of dressings. Taste testing and note-taking is important for when the lettuce porn seed catalogs again arrive in the frozen winter months.

In contrast, in my kitchen, when I think chicories, I think less of delicate leaves and more of delicacy leaves. High cuisine. I think of very special salads like the French *frisée aux lardons*—my version, sans lardons, is given below. And I think of Italian specialties like *insalata tricolore* and *puntarelle alla Romana*. The first, replicating the three colors of the Italian flag, combines arugula, white Belgian endive, and red radicchio, though the latter two seem redundant to me from a family-genus-species perspective. The second is extremely rare, making use of an interesting variety of catalogna that is forced to send up multiple short bolting stems that are harvested at just the right time.

THE ASTER WEEDS: RAGWEED AND GALINSOGA: PRAYING, NOT SPRAYING

The farm is home, unfortunately, to a few very problematic weeds from the Asteraceae family. The dandelions are ubiquitous; annoying, but easy to pull, and rarely causing any serious concern. I occasionally see the pretty blue flowers of common chicory, if we've missed pulling them before they flower. But there is one dreaded Asteraceae weed that I hate to even name: ragweed.

Unlike *Lactuca serriola* (prickly lettuce or milk thistle) and common chicory, ragweed is only distantly related to our Aster Greens, but it is still in the enormous Asteraceae family. I mention it because its objective in life seems to be tearing down and defeating my "great sense of pride and accomplishment" on my farm. Multiple varieties of ragweed exist. Their genus is *Ambrosia*. I seriously don't know why; the name seems so utterly wrong. Its goal is total takeover. Furthermore, it is dreaded not only because its enormous amounts of pollen cause an enormous share of the allergic rhinitis plaguing the country each year (that is, watery eyes, runny noses, and sneezing when the ragweed is in bloom, making billions for big pharma) but also because—unlike the milk thistle, dandelions, and common chicory, which are all pretty easy to suppress with some good old-fashioned weed pulling—ragweed is pernicious. The ragweed plants seem to be sometimes perennial, at other times annual (shooting up from last year's seeds), and, to top it all off, they grow on rhizomes, which are underground stems that send up countless new shoots.

Like the much less concerning lamb's quarters and pig-weed of the Chenopods (which are more neglected super-foods than dreaded weeds), I can spot ragweed from the bottom to the top of a one-hundred-foot bed of vegetables. But unlike other weeds, this weed doesn't just bring a sense of dread; it strikes fear in the heart. Fear of total invasion. This weed is invasive. And I do not use herbicides. I stare it in the stem, blurt several expletives cursing its audacity, and set out on brutal combat, with ungloved hands—ungloved so that I can feel my way along each underground rhizome. My goal is total destruction. Perennially, I win the battle for domination on this farm. This is *my* under-an-acre farm, and the ragweed and other Aster Weeds will not take control.

I had thought that no weed could be more dreaded than ragweed until another Asteraceae weed appeared, expanding its footprint—its foothold—annually, until ultimately it took over entire beds, literally leaving several crops smothered, stunted, and unsalvageable. It's called galinsoga, and it is my worst enemy on the farm, even surpassing ragweed. I cannot discuss it without cursing, inappropriate for a mild-mannered farmer, so I'll say no more about it. Aside from massive amounts of weed pulling and other tricks like tarps, flame weeding, scuffle hoeing, and heavy mulch on my farm, it's about praying, not spraying. No herbicides here. The Aster Greens are clean. I don't even bother to rinse them before making those extraordinarily healthy salads.

Before rising up onto my soapbox, which awaits, I'll just add that most of the Asteraceae plants on the farm are neither the Aster Greens nor the Aster Weeds. They are the glorious flowers that I grow for cutting: Black-eyed Susan (*Rudbeckia*). China asters. Cosmos. Craspedia (sun balls).

Goldenrod. Marigolds. Purple coneflowers and other varieties of echinacea. Sunflowers. Yarrow. Zinnias. And my award-winning dahlias—I won a blue ribbon, a red ribbon, and a white ribbon at the Dutchess County Fair in just my second year of growing them, so, in my mind, they will always be award winning. And, with that, I am hereby admitting, as a grown man with very respectable and frequently commented on biceps, that I absolutely adore flowers, sometimes nearly to the point of tears, especially those within the Aster family.

The Asteraceae family is so large and diverse that even some of our herbs are within the family, like chamomile and tarragon. So is a glorious, delicious delicacy that might occasionally adorn a fancy entrée in a high-end restaurant: sunflower shoots, specialty two-to-three-inch-tall sunflower seedlings. They're actually very easy to grow right in the kitchen, and like other shoots and microgreens, they can make your favorite entrée gourmet. But enough about the Aster Weeds, the Aster Flowers, the Aster Herbs, and the Aster Shoots: our focus here is on the Aster Greens, which leads me to my soapbox about the most grossly overappreciated vegetable of all.

MY ICEBERG SOAPBOX

In some of our eight vegetable family chapters, I home in on some of the most underappreciated vegetables, like kohlrabi within the Brassicas and spinach, beets, beet greens, and Swiss chard within the Chenopods. Here, instead, I harp on about one of the most overappreciated vegetables, even though most people don't really appreciate it at all. Bland, dull, and tasteless—but reliable. Iceberg lettuce.

I've striven, as I write in this old stone house, to reveal myself fully and unabashedly, faults and all, to be completely bare and honest before you—my embarrassing tendency toward crying over stolen cabbage, my feeling ashamed over annual failures with spinach, and, as early as chapter one, my possibly unsavory character trait as an unapologetic vegetable snob. Here, the snobbery peaks, as I speak openly, forcing myself to be ever so brief and to not use dirty words, despite my long-suffering distaste for iceberg lettuce.

Iceberg lettuce. You know, those large, round heads in plastic bags, always piled high in every grocery store. Pale, or even white, inside. Low in nutrients. But high in staying power, being tolerant of weeklong trips in eighteen-wheelers crossing the country from sunny California. Nearly devoid of taste when it leaves and completely devoid when it arrives.

What has happened to us Americans that we so commonly equate lettuce, our countless, glorious *Lactuca sativa* varieties, with iceberg? What has happened, and why, I ask, Socratically, as a vegetable snob?

Well, what has happened is that we have grown to rely on very large growers in select agricultural areas to grow nearly all our vegetables, even nutritionally inferior ones if ideal from a mass-production perspective, so that they are available year-round. This societal culinary failure is exemplified most perfectly by iceberg lettuce. It's easy to grow, easy to harvest, and easy to bag in the field; it boxes well, travels well long distance, and holds up well in the refrigerated nether regions of grocery stores before being brought out and piled high on display. And then it holds up even longer in the home fridge. Yes, it has some vitamin K and vitamin A. And, yes, it has no cholesterol and no fat. And, yes, if you eat enough of it, dropping meat, you'll surely lose weight. But the decisions that went into its packaging and passport properties selected out most of its nutrition and all of its taste.

While the large, tight head of iceberg lettuce in the grocery store might be less expensive than the giant, loose head of MdQS or Merlot that I sell at the farmers market—about two dollars compared to three or four dollars—you get what you pay for, in terms of taste, nutritional value, and impact on the environment. Plus, it's not clear to me how a head of iceberg lettuce can be produced, bagged, boxed, and shipped for two dollars a head, though the large-scale producers have obviously figured it out—and fair labor practices and a living wage might not have been part of the equation.

Iceberg lettuce helped make fast-food restaurants rich and famous, as did unripe tomatoes, which I'll tell you about later. All shredded lettuce in all fast-food chains is iceberg—yet another reason, as if we needed one, to not eat fast food. Glorious, sweet, delicious *Lactuca sativa* has been desecrated.

And cooks and chefs across the country now collectively rely on a special salad that allows them to buy, store, and easily use iceberg lettuce. It's so easy. You quarter it, smother the quarter head in blue cheese dressing (or ranch), sprinkle it with bacon bits or bacon chunks, and throw on a couple of quartered cherry tomatoes to make this "salad" look healthy. Seriously? Even in fancy restaurants? Anything smothered and sprinkled in blue cheese dressing (or ranch) and bacon, respectively, is going to make even the most tasteless leaves taste good. I'd rather have a wedgie than a wedge salad.

Romaine lettuce is also good for large-scale production and transport and, in my view, beats iceberg by only just a bit, mainly because of how delicious Caesar salads can be when prepared really well. My beloved MdQS—the crisp, sweet, delicious, savoyed (curly-leafed) French butterhead lettuce with contrasting pink, red, light green, and dark green leaves—and the gorgeous and delicious Merlot, along with countless other lettuce varieties, don't stand a chance of being loaded into an eighteen-wheeler or piled high in the grocery store. They are too delicate for that, which may be why they are so delicious, primarily during May and early June in my growing zone, and found only at the farmers market or through a CSA.

I now step down from my vegetable snobbery soapbox. I tried to keep it brief. My advice: eat local lettuces from local farms or farmers markets. Advance warning: I'll step back up on the box in our chapter on the beloved Nightshades when I mouth off with yet more snobbery about boring giant green, giant yellow, and giant red bell peppers.

MUSTARDY FRISÉE WITH POACHED EGG, RED RADICCHIO WITH STINKY CHEESE

I previously suggested that *Lactuca sativa* never requires a recipe, though *Cichorium endivia* and *Cichorium intybus* always benefit from one. And since I've previously given my preferred way of preparing white beans with escarole, here I give my favorite chicory salads.

My Mustardy Frisée with Poached Egg. I take a head of frisée, preferably just harvested from the gardens (or just bought at the farmers market), and cut off the lower quarter or so of the head so that the leaves easily fall off. A little more trimming will yield a big bowl of frisée leaves with none of the head's stem. I toss the leaves with my home-made shallot salad dressing (which counts as a second family), though when using it on slightly bitter frisée rather than slightly sweet lettuce, I make the dressing a bit heavier on the honey and the mustard. To this lightly dressed salad, I sprinkle sunflower seeds, as well as salt and pepper to taste. Then, I add homemade croutons and a freshly poached egg (both while still hot, since some minor wilting of the frisée will be just fine). This is my simple version of the French bistro salad frisée aux lardons, but without the lardons (cubed fatty bacon).

I could write a whole book on radicchio, and maybe I will, but here is my favorite way to prepare a freshly cut head of red radicchio.

My Red Radicchio with Stinky Cheese. I take the head of radicchio and slice it into strips the right size for a fork-to-mouth salad. I then take a chunk of soft, stinky blue cheese—whatever looked most interesting and appealing at the grocery store—and scoop up (with my fingers) about two tablespoons, mushing it so that it's creamy on my fingers. I work the cheese across and throughout the sliced radicchio until the red leaves have just the right amount of coverage, adding a bit more cheese if need be. My goal is to have enough of the cheese to balance the bitter radicchio but not so much that the bitterness of the radicchio is completely masked. Then, I add whatever fruit is available (like a thinly sliced pear or quartered figs) and whatever nuts sound good (like walnuts or almond slices). Unlike with other salads, given the diversity of delicious flavors, I abstain from salt and pepper.

During a radicchio-focused tour of the Veneto region of Italy, the motherland of all varieties of radicchio, I made many fond memories of delicious *antipasti*, *primi*, *secondi*, and *contorni* featuring radicchio. One particularly memorable antipasto began with a layer of freshly sliced prosciutto, topped with coarsely sliced radicchio and thinly sliced finocchio (I was in Treviso, not Florence, so I'm hesitant to call it Florence fennel here), and finished with a few sliced figs and the much-required shaved Asiago. Prosciutto! Radicchio! Finocchio! *Buon appetito!*

It's time to turn attention to the bottoms and tops—Florence fennel included—of the Umbellifers.

10.
Apiaceae

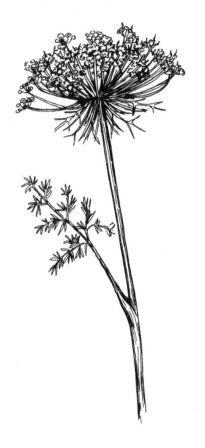

The Umbellifers:

Carrots and Their Cousins, from Bottoms to Tops

CARROTS, PARSNIPS, CELERY, CELERIAC, AND FENNEL, as well as parsley, cilantro, and dill, among other herbs. The Apiaceae family, or Umbelliferae family, includes plants whose defining characteristic is the arrangement of their flowers in umbels, hence their name. What's an umbel? In botany, the term was first used in the 1590s—taken from the Latin *umbella*, meaning "parasol" or "sunshade" (think *umbrella*)—to indicate an inflorescence (cluster of flowers) stemming from a main branch with many smaller branches. In other words, a number of short flower stalks (called pedicels) spread from a common point like the ribs of an umbrella.

That's what the flowers of these flowering plants look like: pretty, lacy, flat umbrellas. But unless we're growing them for seed (or for cut flowers), we usually don't want to see them sending up flowers, as that will ruin the carrot root, fennel bulb, or parsley stems and leaves we're aiming for. I always know that the heat of summer has arrived when my few remaining fennel plants start acting strangely, preparing to send up flowers, splitting the lovely finocchio (Florence fennel) bulbs into tough, inedible, browning segments. Ideally, though, all of it will have been harvested before the bolting would have begun.

As I laid out in chapter one, I now eat carrots, even though I personally had never been a fan and ate them only because I knew that I was supposed to eat them, for my eyes. But I now eat them with delight. And I now eat celery, fennel, and parsley, even though I had never seen a real need for celery (except to add some crunch to tuna salad and the like); I had never eaten fennel, ever; and I had viewed parsley as a garnish and never thought much about it. Things changed when I started growing these Umbellifers. I developed a deep fondness for them: a farmer's fondness for celery, as growing it takes much patience, persistence, and care; and a foodie fondness for carrots, especially the smallish, colorful ones used whole in some of the most savory autumn dishes.

While we eat the seedpods and seeds of the Legumes (except with exceptional treats like alfalfa sprouts, bean sprouts, and pea shoots, when we eat the young plants whole), the leaves of the Aster Greens (except when drinking chicory coffee or chicory tea, in which chicory root is used), and the fruits of the Cucurbits and the Nightshades (except in the case of one strange vegetable that became famous and remains both famous and infamous, which I'll explain), the Umbellifers—like the Brassicas, the Alliums, and the Chenopods— offer us vegetables that may be roots, stems, or leaves. They give us nutrients whether we eat them as a bottom (carrots and parsnips), as a stem (fennel and celery), or as a top (parsley, cilantro, and dill leaves and seeds). This is all a matter of convention; there's no reason why we couldn't or shouldn't eat carrot tops or parsley roots. From bottom to top, they are packed with important nutrients and health-promoting phytonutrients.

CRUNCHY CAROTENE AND OTHER NUTRITION FACTS

Here's the rundown on the Umbellifers' nutritional benefits. Let's start with carrots (*Daucus carota*, subspecies *sativus*). *Sativus*, as you might recall, is Latin for "cultivated," an important distinction, since *Daucus carota* more generally is wild carrot, or the weed called Queen Anne's lace. Specific types of wild carrot were selectively grown over the centuries to produce the carrot qualities that we now take for granted: sweetness instead of bitterness, crunchiness instead of woodiness. Although the stems and leaves are perfectly edible (and quite good in salads and pesto), we usually just eat the carrot's taproot, which contains tons of vitamin A and ample amounts of vitamins K, C, and B6. Carrots are a good source of multiple minerals and have beneficial phytonutrients: purple carrots contain anthocyanins, and orange carrots have alpha- and beta-carotene.

Beta-carotene. It's good for your eyes and good for your skin. Our body converts it into vitamin A, or retinol. It reduces your risk of macular degeneration (think retina). But it's also an antioxidant, helping the immune system and probably reducing our risk of cancer. Although it's named after carrots, beta-carotene is also found in spinach (from the Chenopods), lettuce (from the Aster Greens), winter squash (from the Cucurbits), tomatoes (from the Nightshades), and other veggies.

Next, the carrot's cousin *Pastinaca sativa*, or parsnips—a good source of vitamins K, C, B9 (folate), B6, E, and other micronutrients. More on parsnips later. Now, another cousin of the carrot: celery (*Apium graveolens*). While celery contains fiber and vitamin K and other micronutrients, it is more of a super-ingredient than a superfood. Like the Alliums, in my view, celery makes dishes taste better, and, like the Alliums, we rarely have a side of celery on its own. Any good soup starts with both celery and onion. Celery, from bottom to top, is foundational to many soups, as well as to salads. Bottom refers to celeriac, or the celery root bulb (*Apium graveolens*, variety *rapaceum*), and top to its leaves (as in Chinese leaf celery, *Apium graveolens*, variety *secalinum*) and its seeds (used as a spice).

A word about celeriac, as it is an underappreciated vegetable primarily because many people are completely unfamiliar with it. Despite its strange, knobby, brown appearance, celeriac offers another way of getting the nutritional benefits of the Umbellifers, aside from the more routine celery and carrots. Like celery, it is low in calories and high in fiber, and it's a good source of vitamins C and K, as well as minerals like phosphorus and potassium. In the kitchen, once peeled, celeriac can be grated into salads to add a crisp texture and earthy flavor, with just a hint of celery taste. It can be cooked into soups, stews, and gratins, where its subtle celery-like flavor adds depth and complexity to dishes. In fact, the best celery soup, in my opinion, is made with celeriac (and some potato). Additionally, celeriac can be roasted or puréed to create creamy side dishes or used as a flavorful ingredient in vegetable-based mains, showcasing its adaptability and culinary appeal. And, to top it all, it's relatively easy to grow and keeps very well in the refrigerator or root cellar.

Another carrot cousin: fennel (*Foeniculum vulgare*). Its leaves and seeds are used as flavoring. Florence fennel (finocchio) is a variety with a swollen, bulb-like stem base. A multitude of phytonutrients give it its strong smell and taste (which signals major health benefits), and fennel is a good source of vitamin C and a number of minerals. It may be one of the most studied vegetables in terms of its medicinal properties: aiding digestion and reducing cancer risk and cardiovascular disease risk.

Finally, the "leafy greens" of the Umbellifers, as well as their seeds (like parsley, cilantro, dill, angelica, caraway, and chervil), are undoubtedly healthy and high in micronutrients, though they account for small amounts of our vegetable intake, since they are Umbellifer Herbs. This family of vegetables is not unlike the Alliums in that they make so many of our other vegetables taste so good.

THE SMALL VEGETABLE FARMER'S SEED CATALOG: OP vs. F1

Previously, in the chapter on the Aster Greens, I discussed open pollinated plants and heirlooms—specifically, all the delicious open pollinated varieties of lettuce, a few of which carry the distinction of being heirlooms. Here, with carrots and celery, it's worth mentioning F1, or hybrid, seeds. My farm makes use of a few of these within the Umbellifers but many more in our last two vegetable (fruit) families, the Cucurbits and the Nightshades.

Flipping open my favorite seed catalog, I find two varieties of celery to choose from. One is open pollinated, called Tango (about fourteen dollars for one thousand pelleted seeds); the other is an F1 hybrid called Merengo (about sixteen dollars for one thousand seeds). The latter is available in regular seeds or pelleted seeds; I'll tell you about the difference later. I always grow Tango—not because of the slightly lower cost, but just because it's the one I've always grown, and it tastes great. Merengo probably tastes exactly the same, but as an F1 hybrid, it comes with several added horticultural benefits. It's a bit earlier, ready to harvest after eighty days instead of eighty-five. It's taller, at about twenty-eight inches instead of about twenty. And, most importantly, it has high resistance to fusarium yellows, a soilborne fungus that can infect celery's roots and cause the leaves to turn yellow and brown. The disease has never affected my Tango, so I haven't felt a need to switch to Merengo.

When I flip the page to celeriac, I again find two varieties, one open pollinated and one an F1 hybrid. For parsnips, there are two varieties, both open pollinated, and, for Florence fennel, we have one open pollinated variety and four hybrid types. I assume the hybrids provide for larger, more reliable bulbs and better bolt resistance.

But when I flip back to the carrots, always up near the front of the catalogs, I'm met with not just a couple of varieties but eighteen. Carrots are beloved by all small farmers—delightful to CSA members, beautiful in bunches piled high at the farmers market, and delicious when roasted with some honey from right here on the farm. Some varieties are short and pudgy, others long and sharply pointed, and a few are in non-orange colors: white, yellow, red, and purple. Among this catalog's nineteen particular cultivars, six are hybrids, eight are open pollinated, and two are deemed heirlooms (the Red Cored Chantenay and Danvers 126, both of which probably have a lengthy provenance, which I haven't looked into because I don't grow them, opting instead for my own rainbow blend, as I'll describe).

Unlike the lettuces, among the Umbellifers and many of the other families we have F1 hybrid seeds among our options. Here's how F1 hybrids work. One specific variety of, in this case, open pollinated carrot is crossbred—or "cross-fertilized" or "cross-pollinated"—with another specific variety of open pollinated carrot. Rather than producing carrots characteristic of the first or second variety, a new variety of carrot is created. Maybe it combines the sweet flavor of the first with the disease tolerance of the second, or the healthy and durable tops of one (good for pulling and bunching) with the uniformity in shape of the other. When those new plants' seeds are sown the next season, we once again get the great new carrot cultivar. It usually has a terrific name that is featured prominently in the carrot porn section of the seed catalog.

Unlike with open pollinated seeds, though, if we were to try our hand at seed saving, it wouldn't work so well. F1 hybrid seeds do not breed true, so we can't pass the seeds down through the generations from one granny to the next. These F1 seeds need to be made by the seed companies year after year. (If the F1 plants are allowed to self-pollinate, the resulting seed would be F2, or second generation, though they would lack the vigor and consistency of the designer F1 generation.)

The seed companies provide us with these wonderful varieties, which are created under controlled conditions. While it's technical, crossbreeding is not unnatural. For example, if you plant a number of varieties of open pollinated summer squash in close proximity, eat and enjoy them, but inadvertently leave one behind in the garden, with a seed from it germinating in the spring, you might very well have created for yourself some strange new squash varieties. (That doesn't happen with carrots, however, as we never see them flower and produce pollen, since they are biennials and would flower only in their second year.) Such a squash was created in my garden one year, an F1 hybrid from Mother Nature rather than from my own controlled cross-pollination, and I thought that I might become rich and famous for the strange but very delicious new variety. I didn't. I'll tell you about it when we get to the Cucurbits.

GROWING CARROTS ON MY LITTLE FARM, AND NOT GROWING PARSNIPS BECAUSE MY FARM IS LITTLE

When I first started growing vegetables at a small scale but in a "production" mode, among the many dozens of vegetables, my two least favorite to grow were carrots and celery—not because I hadn't yet begun developing a fondness for eating and sharing them with others, but because at first they seemed hard to grow. Carrots are difficult because once the tiny seeds are directly sown into the garden (which is difficult itself, as the seeds are so very tiny, which is why pelleted seeds are so amazing), they are slow to germinate. It can take two full weeks before the tiny cotyledons begin emerging, and usually by then the weed seeds have readily germinated and have nearly taken over the bed. It thus becomes difficult to remove the weeds while sparing the tiny carrot seedlings. Every year, I learn more about growing carrots.

Celery has also vied for my least favorite vegetable to grow, mainly, again, because of how slow it is to germinate indoors. Celery seeds, while looking much like carrot seeds, are sown not into the garden soil directly but, in my case at least, into a 1020 tray indoors. Rather than using seventy-two-cell 1020 flats, I use a 1020 tray and "broadcast" sow the celery seeds, eventually ending up with many hundreds of seedlings that will be potted up. Celery is the first vegetable that I seed, usually on February 26 or so. More than two months later, and after having been "pricked out" and potted up, they get transplanted into the garden, also a difficult task, as they are delicate—delicate and fussy. But within a couple more months, these plants become worth the fuss.

Now, since becoming enthusiastic about eating my own carrots and my own celery—and about growing these vegetables for others to delight in—I view their cultivation to be an annual ritual challenge for my green thumbs, pushing myself to improve further each year. And now, having heard from farmers market shoppers and CSA members, "Your celery is the best I've ever eaten!" and "Your carrots are so delicious!" the reward is worth the challenges.

I understand each of these cousins quite well. As expected, the carrots, celery, fennel, and parsley cousins have quite a bit in common. Their seeds have similarities, and their seedlings, when less than a couple inches tall, are virtually identical. I can only tell the difference between an inch-tall celery plant and an inch-tall parsley plant by eating it. That's why labels are helpful in the first few weeks in the greenhouse.

Even though I don't often see their flowers on the farm, the Apiaceae have lovely, lacy, fanciful flowers. Thanks to those flowers, I can look at a weed/wildflower both here in the United States or when travelling abroad and know when I'm looking at yet another Umbellifer cousin, a distant, wild relative of the carrots and fennel. Queen Anne's lace, a weed that I try to keep out of my gardens, is simply, as I noted, a wild carrot. Since the flower itself didn't convince me during my first year of farming (though it should have, being a classic Apiaceae flower), I pulled up the taproot and took a bite. And then spit it out. Yep, that's a wild carrot alright. It'll make you appreciate the *sativus* cultivars.

For my carrots, I select five varieties—not caring if they're open pollinated or F1 hybrid—that come in pelleted seeds and that give me the full array of carrot colors: white, yellow, orange, red, and purple. And I make sure they're all described in the seed catalog as being ready to harvest right around the same time, at about seventy days (as opposed to some being fifty-five to sixty-five and others eighty to ninety-five). I blend the seeds and sow them in four long rows per thirty-inch bed, and when it's time to harvest, I pull them up by the handful, resulting in gorgeous rainbow bundles ready to be rinsed and loaded into the van for the farmers market. Given my tight dimensions, that bed is then immediately prepared and replanted, often with green beans, which is good for the soil.

I'm a big fan of pelleted carrot seeds. Regular carrot seeds are very, very tiny. When sowing the regular carrot seeds in my four long rows, it's very hard to space them about two inches apart. Sometimes multiple seeds fall into the same cranny in the soil. Those carrots, if not thinned as seedlings (which would be excessively tedious unless growing just a short row), might well produce taproots that are underdeveloped because they've had insufficient space to grow. With pelleted seeds, I can easily sow one about every two inches and never have to think about overcrowding.

What is pelleted seed? Pelleting is just for very small seeds. Those tiny seeds are coated with an inert, dissolvable material, like a clay mixture, to give them a larger, round, smooth, uniform shape and size. Perfectly easy to work with. They were really developed for commercial growers who use machines to sow seeds, allowing for better accuracy of the seeder in spacing. The only other family for which I seek out pelleted seed is the Aster Greens. Lettuce seeds are equally tiny, but when it's pelleted seed going into the seventy-two cells of a 1020 flat, it's like sowing Tic Tacs. The only drawbacks are that pelleted seeds are a bit more expensive, and they don't keep well from one season to the next.

Why so much talk about carrots and carrot seeds and carrot flowers with such little mention of their cousin the parsnips? I've had farm customers ask for a produce item that I hadn't been growing, and the next year I would set out to grow it. Small, local farmers love doing this. It's how I got started with escarole a few years ago. And then one thing led to another, and I found myself growing every chicory I could find, catalogna (Italian dandelion) included. I've always grown carrots on the farm, as they are a staple that everyone delights in. I've been waiting for a customer to ask me for parsnips, in which case I might well feel the need to give my green thumbs a try at them. But none yet has, and thus I have yet to do so. Admittedly, I'm a bit ashamed that I've never grown parsnips.

I'm ambivalent about parsnips—an unapologetic vegetable snob ambivalent about parsnips. I had never bought them in the grocery store until this writing in this cold month, when I felt that any respectable farmer and doctor writing about vegetables, and the Umbellifers in particular, should be an expert in parsnips. I'm not. But I did buy a few and made a couple dishes with them. Tasty. It was my first entrée into the small world of parsnips. I had only ever eaten them as a fancy purée alongside a fancy entrée in a fancy restaurant. Good, but not better than carrots. They are indeed a great winter root vegetable for roasting and soups. But I have not yet been convinced to grow them.

Why so much hesitation about growing parsnips? The main problem is one of real estate. It's about fast growers versus slow growers. My beautiful bunches of rainbow carrots are ready for roasting in just seventy days after sowing. Parsnips? They take one hundred twenty days at least, potentially much longer. That's at least four full months compared to less than two and a half. Yes, I'm impatient, but I also need to reuse my beds. For the same reason, when I'm selecting my cabbage seeds from the seed catalog, I pick those ready in sixty to seventy days over those needing one hundred to 125. As soon as the early summer cabbage is harvested, beets or the like are sown behind. Carrots out, green beans in. Veggies best grown in the spring to be harvested in the late spring and early summer are followed by veggies best grown in the summer to be harvested in late summer and early fall.

HONEY ROASTED CARROTS, PARSLEY-WALNUT PESTO

I've hinted a few times at eating ambrosia in the form of honey roasted carrots. The "added sugar" from my honey doesn't concern me given that cooked carrots are probably healthier than raw ones—cooking makes more beta-carotene available to our bodies. Here's how I do it.

My Honey Roasted Carrots. I cut off the carrot tops, saving them for a batch of carrot-top pesto the next day, and wash the carrots well because I'm not going to peel them (the skins might well be the healthiest part). Rather than slicing them into bite-sized coins, I quarter them lengthwise.

I place them in a roasting pan with low walls so that they're just touching but not on top of one another. I drizzle them with a mixture of one-part olive oil and one-part honey (a couple tablespoons of each) and sprinkle with salt and pepper. Or a little cayenne pepper if I want some heat. Or some other favored spice, whether it be thyme, oregano, or the carrots' cousin coriander. Or some freshly cut herbs, like chervil, cilantro, dill, chopped fennel fronds, or parsley (I am not at all opposed to combining Umbellifer Vegetables with Umbellifer Herbs, despite it counting as only one family). Then they go into the oven at 400 degrees Fahrenheit for about thirty to forty minutes until they are just the right tenderness. Or at 425 degrees Fahrenheit for about twenty-five. Or a little higher and a little shorter, or a little lower and a little longer. Until tender. That's it. No recipe required. Ambrosia.

Parsnips? Ditto. Honey roasted parsnips.

I make a lot of pesto, which I mainly use with pasta, though it's also good for drizzling on salads, sides, and entrées, quiches and pizzas included. I make traditional basil pesto, plus stranger ones like carrot-top pesto, but my favorite pesto is with parsley (and with walnuts rather than pine nuts)—perfect for catching up on my Umbellifers if I've missed out on carrots, celery, and the like for a day or two. Pesto is quick and easy if you have a basic kitchen food processor. It's especially delicious when the parsley (or basil, or carrot tops, or arugula) is straight from the gardens or the farmers market.

My Parsley-Walnut Pesto. I take out the food processor and prepare all my ingredients. Then, it's only about two minutes of work until the pesto is ready for the pasta. I start by placing about two cups of slightly packed, coarsely chopped flat Italian parsley into the food processor bowl. Then, I add about a third of a cup of chopped walnuts, about a third of a cup of grated parmesan, and salt and pepper to taste. I pulse the food processor several times until the parsley is finely chopped and the ingredients well mixed. I take a spatula and wipe down the sides of the food processor bowl. Then, with about a third of a cup of extra virgin olive oil ready, I turn the food processor on and slowly pour in the oil, watching carefully for consistency. Once it gets to the perfect pesto consistency, I turn off the food processor, and it's done. I follow the exact same process and amounts for a pesto of basil and pine nuts, a pesto of arugula and almonds, and a pesto of carrot tops and pistachios—in essence, whatever pesto-enticing green is on the farm and whatever pesto-compatible nuts are in the pantry.

11.

Cucurbitaceae

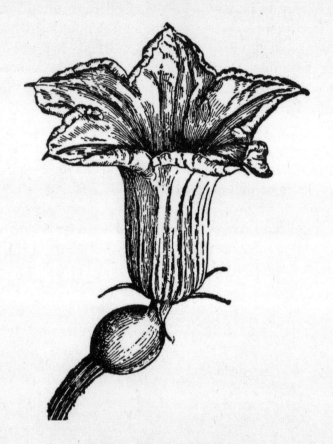

The Cucurbits:

Fruit Vegetables (or Vegetable Fruits) for Every Season

THIS MIGHT WELL BE MY FAVORITE FAMILY AMONG
THE EIGHT, though I might have said that before. I've put
the Cucurbits at number seven not because I don't absolutely love cucumbers, summer squash, melons, watrmelons,
and winter squash but because their nutritional value, while
very good, doesn't rival that of the Brassicas and some of the
other superfoods. The Cucurbitaceae family includes herbaceous plants (and a few very rare shrubs), usually vining
rampantly on the ground or else climbing about using spiral
tendrils. What's a tendril? It's a specialized curly stem with
a threadlike shape used by a number of climbing plants for
support and attachment in twining around suitable hosts,
like another plant, a tree trunk, my cucumber trellises, or my
pea trellises. The plant's tendrils—whether the Legumes, the
Cucurbits, or others—find their hosts, like a nearby bush or
my fence-like trellises, by touch perception. The biology is
not only intricately complex but a masterpiece of evolution-
ary engineering.

But tendrils, albeit important for some of the Cucurbits,
are not the part of the plant we're usually most attentive to.
It's their flowers—big, beautiful, inviting yellow or orange
flowers. The Cucurbits have unisexual flowers, with male
and female flowers on the same plant. The male flowers
produce the pollen. The female flowers have an ovary that
swells into a fruit, full of seeds. All the Cucurbit vegetables
are, in fact, fruits. We usually don't eat any of their roots or
stems or leaves, just their fruits. These vegetables are fruits
horticulturally but vegetables culinarily (except for the melons and watermelons, which are fruits culinarily because of
their sugar content).

Among the nearly one thousand species across multiple genera within the Cucurbitaceae family, I am interested—since this is a story about my vegetables—in only three such genera. There are others that are edible, including species providing fruits that are more relevant outside of the United States and that I have never grown, like bitter melons, caigua, and calabash, but I'm focusing on those that we all know best: *Cucumis*, or cucumbers, cantaloupes, and honeydews; *Cucurbita*, or summer squash, winter squash, and pumpkins; and *Citrullus*, or watermelons.

Here on the farm, I find the Cucurbits to be fun to grow in several ways. First, they have big seeds (think about cucumber seeds, watermelon seeds, pumpkin seeds, and so on), which are, in contrast to those of the Brassicas, the Aster Greens, and the Umbellifers, easy and fun to sow into our seed flats. Compared to the big seeds of the Legumes (which are round like peas or oval like pinto beans), the Cucurbits' seeds are equally big, but they're flat, containing the two large cotyledons just waiting to burst forth with life within a few days of sowing.

I use 1020 flats with fifty cells for this and only this family, rather than the seventy-two-cell flats that I use for most of the other families. Why? Well, that's the second reason why the Cucurbits are fun to grow: the seedlings are big and robust, growing quickly (and thus benefiting from the extra rooting space in the fifty-cell flats before being transplanted out). Third, they are fun because once transplanted out, they again grow quickly, some getting viny and wanting to climb all over everything around them, soon displaying their big male and female flowers, which are almost immediately distinguishable because the female flowers have a rapidly growing fruit at their base. This is where the honeybees and bumblebees pitch in on the farm: free labor. Finally, growing the Cucurbits is fun because the plants and their fruits are fun to watch grow, and the harvest is fun and gratifying. If you've ever grown your own zucchini (you only need a few plants for a bountiful harvest), you know what I mean.

THE CUCURBITS IN THREE GENEROUS GENERA: CUCUMIS, CUCURBITA, AND CITRULLUS

First, *Cucumis.*

Cucumbers are of the genera *Cucumis sativus.* The cucumber fruits are produced on vines that use tendrils to figure out where to grow without strangling themselves. If grown on the ground, the tendrils wrap themselves around the sturdiest weed they can find, and their fruits are mostly hidden by their leaves, making the harvest all the more fun. Many grocery store cucumbers are grown with much more sophistication and technology than I have on my little plot, like special cultivars that are "parthenocarpic," meaning that the flowers do not require pollination and yield mostly seedless fruit, all done on trellis wires in massive greenhouses. I grow mine on a regular fence-like trellis, or, even more commonly, just on the ground.

There are countless varieties of cucumbers for growers to choose from, generally falling into the categories of slicing, pickling, gherkin, and burpless, the latter seedless and with more delicate and thin skin, thus "easier to digest" (read: less burping)—though I've never had a problem digesting cucumbers. Some people are prone to burping after eating cucumbers, and it evidently comes from a phytochemical called cucurbitacin, which is highest in the stems, skin, and seeds. One might speculate that the cucurbitacin is some sort of defense mechanism; maybe if the cucumber beetles are busy burping, they'll eat less. I don't know anything else about cucumber-induced burping. The farting lecture in medical school was quick and embarrassing, but the burping lecture was even more abrupt and transitory, with no mention of cucumbers.

Cucumbers have a little sugar, a little fiber, a little protein, and negligible fat. They are generally low in micronutrients, though they do have some vitamin K. In my mind, they qualify as very healthy not because they are packed with vitamins, minerals, and beneficial phytonutrients but because they taste good and make us more likely to eat a salad.

Related to *Cucumis sativus* is *Cucumis melo*, the melons. Here, the fruits are sweeter—so much so that we treat them, when we eat them, like fruit. But on the farm, growing melons is like growing cucumbers, except for the art and science of when to pick the melons. Because we eat melons for their sugar content, they have to be harvested at just the right time, which is one of the biggest melon challenges for home gardeners. Picked too early, a melon will probably taste more like a cucumber. Although grocery stores usually have just cantaloupes and honeydews, there are numerous cultivars of melons, many of which are juicy, delicious, mouth-watering heirlooms. Delicious 51, Fordhook Gem, Noir des Carmes, Prescott Fond Blanc, Pride of Wisconsin, and countless others. The melons have some vitamin A and some vitamin C. Like eating cucumbers, you cannot get fat by eating too many of them; they're mostly water.

Second, *Cucurbita*.

I love this genus. The *Cucurbita* are the squashes, native to the Americas but beloved around the world. *Cucurbita* come in just a few species; I am familiar with three: *Cucurbita pepo*, *Cucurbita maxima*, and *Cucurbita moschata*. In most basic farming terms, they are summer squash when picked still young and tender with thin, edible skin (mostly the *pepo*); they are winter squash, on the other hand, when allowed to stay on the vine until it starts to die and the fruits' skins are hard, making the fruits storable. Some varieties are specifically grown to be summer squash, and others to be fall or winter squash. *Cucurbita pepo* alone gives us yellow summer squash (both crookneck and straightneck, or, to be more fun and interesting, *torticollis* and *recticollis*), zucchini, and pattypan, but also acorn squash, delicata squash, spaghetti squash, and even pumpkins. Like the cucumbers and melons, the squashes give us some sugars and a few vitamins, but here we get even more fiber, especially from the winter squash.

While these fruits might not be superfoods, pepitas or pumpkin seeds, on the other hand, do qualify. They are—obviously—not mostly water; they are high in fiber, healthy fats, and protein; and they are replete with vitamins and minerals. They're great in lieu of bacon bits on any salad. I always have pumpkin seeds in the pantry for salads; just a few transform any salad from bland to gourmet. And pepitas are a key ingredient in my homemade trail mix. All of that healthy fat and protein will keep you going whether you're climbing a mountain, weeding the carrots, or stuck at the desk.

Third, *Citrullus*.

The delicious watermelon is *Citrullus lanatus*. Why is a story about vegetables mentioning watermelon, since we all know it, clearly, as fruit? Well, if we're going to call cucumbers and zucchini—and tomatoes, peppers, and eggplants—vegetables, then we're going to cover watermelons in this story about vegetables, too.

Just as cucumbers, melons, and squash are ancient, so too are watermelons. They were at one time grown in arid regions because they could be stored and eaten during the dry seasons as a source of food as well as water. That makes sense, because, as its name implies, watermelon is mostly water, with some sugar (which is why we love it), and a little vitamin C. Not much else in terms of nutritional value, but so refreshing on a hot August afternoon.

There are hundreds of varieties of watermelons—not just the giant striped ones in the huge boxes at the grocery store that provide a decent workout by simply lifting one into the buggy. Black Diamond Yellow Belly. Cream of Saskatchewan. Crimson Sweet. Georgia Rattlesnake. Klondike Blue Ribbon Striped. Little Darling. Orange Tendersweet. Sugar Baby. Yellow Petite. And so many others. There's a sacred text that catalogues and details them that was written just across the river from here.

TWO CUCURBIT BIBLES FROM ACROSS THE RIVER

My little farm is situated on the west side of the Hudson River in Ulster County, just 3.5 miles as the crow flies, to the river, or 5.6 miles via our winding roads. Just across that river, in Dutchess County, a land of many other farms, is a farm much larger than mine. On that farm, perhaps also with an old stone house, though I don't know, another mental health professional embraced a life-changing calling to grow vegetables: Amy Goldman, or Amy Goldman Fowler—an idol of mine given her passion for gardening, growing a huge diversity of cultivars, and seed saving. I've never met her, but I've read two of the Cucurbit bibles she wrote. Those bibles make the seed catalogs look like soft porn. They're both full of gorgeous centerfolds cover to cover.

The Compleat Squash: A Passionate Grower's Guide to Pumpkins, Squashes and Gourds covers some 150 varieties from their seeds to their cured fruits that will store for months. The Melon—as well as her earlier Melons for the Passionate Grower: With Practical Advice on Growing, Pollinating, Picking, and Preparing an Extraordinary Harvest—covers more than one hundred mouthwatering melon and watermelon varieties. Very nerdy stuff, but Cucurbit canons for gardeners and farmers alike.

SELECTING THIS YEAR'S CUCURBITS

In growing these fruits, it might appear that the process doesn't begin until early May, when we spend a half day—or two full days if it's that strange year when nearly the whole farm is dedicated to winter squash—dropping the large, flat seeds into their cells, one flat of fifty, another flat of fifty, another flat of fifty, and so on. But the process actually starts in December, when, with seed catalogues and the two Cucurbit bibles on hand, I make next year's cultivar selections.

For the cucumbers, my favorite seed catalog has twenty-seven varieties to choose from, all organic-certified seeds. Many of these are F1 hybrid varieties that are especially suited to growing under protection (trellised in greenhouses), where they are sheltered from rain and thus from rain splattering soil and many of the soilborne diseases to which cucumbers are so prone onto their leaves.

However, I grow my cucumbers outside in the fresh air and the rain, and I rely on the honeybees and bumblebees to help make it happen—the old-fashioned way as opposed to parthenocarpic plants grown in protected culture. It worked for Granny, and it works for me. But I'm just trying to supply CSA members and farmers market customers, not an entire grocery store chain.

In addition to occasionally trying a few F1 hybrid cucumber varieties—efforts that didn't bring much added benefit to my little farm—I've tried a few of the heirloom varieties: Suyo Long, a Chinese heirloom; lemon cucumbers, which are supposed to look like lemons, though mine looked like brown lemons; and Boothby's Blonde, which was deemed by farm members to be too seedy. Too much burping, I guess.

And I've tried a few special open pollinated cucumber varieties, like Diva, a perfect five-to-seven-inch, thin-skinned, mouthwatering cucumber. It's what I prefer. Or Manny, which is also a perfect five to seven inches but an F1 hybrid. Despite the specialty options, my farm members wanted just a basic cucumber. Your regular, durable, eight-to-nine-inch variety. They don't want basic carrots, basic lettuce, or basic tomatoes, but they do want basic cucumbers.

I've settled into growing one very reliable producer, called Marketmore 76. It's your basic, standard cucumber, probably the one that's piled high in grocery stores. As a vegetable snob, I write this with a sliver of shame and embarrassment—the only time I use "basic" to describe my otherwise "gourmet" produce.

With that easy selection made, the summer squash pose a bit more of a challenge. I'll need a yellow squash, a zucchini, and a pattypan. Here, I'm looking for reliability, disease resistance, and good looks. For the yellow squash, I lean toward recticollis over torticollis, for two reasons. One reason is reasonable; the other is not. First, I find the straight-necked varieties easier to work with in the kitchen. That's because I eat most of my yellow squash fried. Yes, I'm a doctor writing about healthy eating, and I have just admitted to eating fried food. I'm just being honest. (I'll share my recipe shortly.) Second, I've only ever had one trip to the emergency room in which opioids and benzodiazepines were urgently needed. It was some sort of idiopathic "torticollis," as it's called (twisted neck), caused by a neck strain, and it was a serious pain in the neck. So, I don't like even the thought of "torticollis," yellow squash included. I know, it's unreasonable. But that's how trauma works.

For the zucchini, I look back through my past years' notes to select ones (and deselect others) based on productivity and disease resistance. Unlike the winter squash varieties with a range of flavors, zucchini tastes like zucchini, and I just want a lot of them, whether open pollinated or F1 hybrid. For the pattypan (grown not for any unique taste, since it tastes to me like zucchini, but for its unique and funny shape), I usually go with the Bennings Green Tint heirloom.

Choosing the winter squash is even more complicated on my little farm. Once again, the options are endless. Reading the descriptions, I look at days to harvest (there's a big difference between ninety days and 115 days, especially when the beetles are even hungrier than I am). I look at viral disease resistance. I look at expected weight of the finished fruit. I look at full-vining versus partial-bush plant habitus. I look at overall appearance of the fully cured fruit (since it'll be visible on the countertop or in the cellar for many months), in search of glorious grays and glamorous stripes. While I admire the strange heirlooms and outrageous shapes of winter squash that Amy across the river so thoroughly documented, I need something that farm customers are going to want to roast and eat: smooth texture and great taste. I usually go with just two varieties—a butternut and a delicata—due to space constraints. Because of their viny nature, winter squash takes up a lot of space. It also takes a lot of time, and I won't be able to reuse the beds they're in.

Several of my Cucurbits each year are F1 hybrid varieties. I've never set about trying to create hybrids myself here on my farm like the seed companies do. But once upon a time, Mother Nature did, right here in my garden. And I thought it might make me rich. And famous.

RICH AND FAMOUS HERE IN MY GARDEN. NOT.

I once thought that I had inadvertently created (Mother Nature was the actual creator) an F1 hybrid that might just make me rich and famous. It was a number of years ago in my original garden, the size of the garage and beside the garage, before I started growing for others. I had several varieties of *Cucurbita pepo* growing, including a yellow torticollis squash (despite my usual objections), a zucchini, another summer squash, and some sort of acorn squash. They're all within the same species and so can cross-pollinate, but they're obviously quite different in shape and taste and thus a bit different genetically. They were planted in very close proximity, obviously with no barrier to the cross-pollination that occurred every time the breeze blew through or the bees buzzed in. They were all delicious fruits. But I evidently left one behind in the garden, probably hidden underneath a dying acorn squash vine, otherwise I would've eaten it.

That fully mature, decaying fruit remained in the garden, full of large, flat seeds. In the spring, one of those seeds, which had hardly but hardily survived the long winter, germinated. By the time I was weeding the newly planted garden in the spring, the squash plant (a weed) was too big for me to, with any love in my heart, pull out and toss into the wheelbarrow, even though it met all criteria for being a weed—the main one simply being an unplanted plant growing in the wrong place. Granny used to call these weeds from last year's vegetables "volunteers," so I do too. I let the volunteer squash plant grow.

Much to my surprise, the volunteer produced a bounty of very strange fruit—strange not in shape, as they resembled a typical mildly crooknecked summer squash, but in coloring. They were light yellow from the top of the neck to three-fourths of the way down, at which point the color changed abruptly, on a straight line dissecting the fruit, from light yellow to a light, pale green. All of them.

They were strange and fabulous—strange in coloring, not in taste, as they tasted like yellow summer squash prepared, as usual, in my frying pan.

I knew enough to know that I could save these F1 hybrid seeds and get the same fruit again next year. But I also knew that I did not know the specifics of the parental lineages needed to reproduce the strange fruit in subsequent years. I hadn't even saved the little plastic markers from the four packs of seedlings I had planted the year prior. But, surely, somehow, I could figure this out. The stakes were high. This could be a whole new summer squash invention. My own cultivar. A game changer that could make me into a legitimate botanist once and for all.

I took pictures of this fabulous new F1 fruit. I texted them around to friends, suggesting that the new variety might soon grace the seed catalogs as Michael's Bicolor Crookneck. I was proud. And eager for the fame. Some friends texted back to congratulate me while, unbeknownst to me, undoubtedly rolling their eyes. Others just rolled their eyes, not offering a response. And, alas, yet another doused my high-flung hopes with a simple, non-congratulatory text back:

"OMG Ive seen those at the farmers market LOL"

No punctuation. Just doused hopes.

The shameful walk from vegetable garden to laptop then commenced for a Google entry of "strange squash that is half yellow and half green." My newly invented squash immediately appeared in beautiful images: Zephyr (F1) squash, "a hybrid squash developed in 1999 by Rob Johnson of Johnny's Seeds." It's "easily distinguished by its slender crooked shape and its signature two-toned appearance. Its stem end carries a faded yellow color while its blossom end is dipped in a pale lime green."

This Rob had beaten me to it. And I'm sure he had put much more effort into it than my serendipity—or, I should say, Mother Nature's smarts—had.

I was obviously disheartened. But, ultimately, I'm more interested in growing (and eating) squash than I am in making F1 hybrid seeds, so I fried the fruit, ate too much, and got over it.

PESTS AND A HIGHER POWER: PRAYING, NOT SPRAYING

By early May, all the Cucurbit seeds have been meticulously selected and we've seeded them into the fifty-cell 1020 flats in the greenhouse as we start the journey toward producing these delightful and delicious fruits. I've suggested that growing these fruits is so much fun, from the initial sowing of the large, flat seeds to the thrill of the harvest. The downside, however, is that at each step of the way, for this family perhaps more than any of the other seven, we are met with a series of problems and pests, from vermin to viruses.

There are four steps that I follow to address these challenges. Step 1 of saving the Cucurbits from an early demise is about the mice—or the mouse.

I never see mice on my little farm, but I know they are around in early May because they seek out one, or actually two, delicious and nutritious types of food: cucurbit seeds and sunflower seeds. I can have forty seed flats on tables made of wood pallets, either in the greenhouse or outside in the elements, with not-yet-germinated seeds and seedlings alike, across all eight families, and the mice, or mouse, seek out just these two: cucurbit seeds and sunflower seeds. I have to cover the fifty-cell flats of freshly sown cucumber, melon, summer squash, winter squash, and watermelon seeds with clear plastic humidity domes, not to keep the humidity in but to keep the despicable vermin out. Without those humidity domes, weighted down with leftover lumber and a few select rocks, each of those fifty seeds, sown about an inch under the soil, in each of those 1020 flats, will be gone by sunrise. The pepitas (pumpkin seeds) are nutritious superfoods not just for us but, evidently, also for rodents.

Once germinated after a successful step 1, the large seedlings grow quickly, and the mice (or mouse) become completely uninterested. The big seedlings require some love and nurturance, but they are usually vigorous and eager for their own piece of this farm. They won't get it, however, until it's hot. They, along with the Nightshades, as we'll see, like the heat of summer. They must not be planted out too early, before the soil is warm, the days long, and the air hot. As such, they have a special place in my heart, as I, too, am a heat-loving organism. (But they don't just get depressed by the first frost in October; rather, unlike the Brassicas, the Chenopods, and some others, they die altogether.) These plants probably originated in subtropical, temperate climates, and Mother Nature did not design them to tolerate a frost. Maybe the biotech companies are working on it. Thus, step 2 of saving the Cucurbits from an early demise is about not planting them out too early, before the threat of a final, unexpected frost lifts—or even before the soil is warm enough.

Step 2 accomplished, the growing begins. They grow well, and they grow quickly. They flower early, and those flowers (the female ones) set fruit readily. All this growth, however, assumes that they don't get decimated by one disease or another. Some years, I have a patch of cucumbers or zucchini that develop some sort of disease, turn brown, dry up, and die. As a nerdy farmer, I'm supposed to look it up and figure it out, with prevention in mind for next year. But plant diseases have yet to pique my interest, and my crop loss each year is minor. I pull out the plants that succumbed to disease, sow some beans, and move on, hoping that rotation will do the job.

Compared to the plants in the other families, the Cucurbits have lots of diseases: downy mildew; bacterial wilt; fusarium wilt; anthracnose; cucumber mosaic virus; squash mosaic virus; watermelon mosaic virus. The list goes on. It's as bad as the tomato blights.

Step 3 of saving the Cucurbits is hoping that rotation worked and that Mother Nature is merciful. Rotation means that a bed is planted in Brassicas one year but not the next. Maybe Alliums the next. And then the Chenopods. And then the Cucurbits. On a compact farm, it never works out quite right because I only have so many beds, they are all close to one another, and I need more space for some families (like the Brassicas and the Cucurbits) than I do for others (like the Chenopods, which are just beets and Swiss chard, since I can't grow spinach). Rotation is more about practical planning than a science, at least with my tight dimensions. But I rotate the best I can to reduce all of these Cucurbit diseases from emerging even more voraciously next year.

Step 4 of saving the Cucurbits is more spiritual than the practical nature of humidity domes, avoiding late frosts, and crop rotation. It's about acknowledging that the inevitable will most likely arrive and praying to a higher power that the very gods who inspired the Cucurbit bibles from across the river will have mercy, that my plants will be robust enough to withstand the trials and tribulations.

This step 4 threat? Cucumber beetles—all sorts of bugs. Striped ones. Spotted ones. Mostly yellow ones. Mostly brown ones. Odorless ones. Stinky ones. They don't necessarily bother the Cucurbit flowers or the emerging fruits (though some do), but they do bother the leaves, those giant Cucurbit leaves that are the power plants of our fruiting operation.

Many or most normal farms (or I should use the proper but really bad term "conventional farms," as opposed to organic) would spray pesticides at this point. An easy step 4 solution. My small-scale farm philosophy, though, is to pray, not spray. I fearfully but faithfully let the bugs run their course chowing down on the Cucurbit leaves with the hope that the plants will be victorious. Some years the farm is nearly free of them. I don't know why. But most years, the destruction begins, the plants' growth slows drastically, the beetles and bugs finish their life cycle, and the plants recover and take off again, shocked and awed but ready to rally until our bushel baskets are overflowing and I'm feeling rich and famous inside, without the dollars or the notoriety to show for it.

FRIED SUMMER SQUASH, ROASTED WINTER SQUASH

Nothing says spring like the bounty of yellow squash and zucchini featured in the first few CSA farm shares. It means I've succeeded across all four steps, even though, to the farm customers, I made it seem easy. And nothing says summer like a cool, crunchy cucumber, or a big slice of watermelon on either side of the river, Amy's Moon and Stars or my Yellow Petite. And nothing says fall and winter like roasted delicata and roasted butternut—or buttercup, which might be my favorite. These are the vegetable fruits that delight us across every season.

I was raised on fried squash, whether at our own kitchen table or across the gardens at Granny's. It's easy, and there are endless variations to the process. Here's my basic approach.

My Fried Summer Squash. I slice the yellow squash (or zucchini) at just the right thickness. It takes trial and error, but I aim for about a quarter of an inch. On a plate, I whisk two eggs. A squirt of mustard whisked in will add some interesting flavor. In another dish, I prepare a mixture of corn meal, flour, and panko (or just one or two of those) and season it with salt and pepper. I heat a thin layer of oil (like olive or grape-seed oil) in a large skillet. I'm not going to "deep fry" the squash, so just a layer of oil of less than a quarter of an inch or so does the trick. I dredge each squash slice through the egg and mustard, then through the corn meal mix, and I fry it until one side is golden brown, flipping to do the same for the other. I always make extra so that I'll have enough for breakfast, since fried squash is one of my drugs of choice.

I, for some reason, was not raised on roasted winter squash. I'm not sure why we didn't grow it in our garden or in Granny's. But I readily acquired the taste for it in adulthood. And it vies with the ambrosia of honey roasted carrots—but instead of honey, I prefer maple syrup. Again, there are countless variations, but the basic idea is as follows.

My Roasted Winter Squash. I quarter the squash, careful not to amputate one or more fingers. I use a small knife to remove the seeds, leaving only the firm meat. Then, I slice the wedge into about one-inch strips and toss them with a mixture of half olive oil and half maple syrup. I sprinkle with salt, pepper, and whatever spice interests me that night, even a little cayenne pepper if I'm feeling spicy. I roast in a pan with low walls at about 425 degrees Fahrenheit for about twenty minutes, flip the pieces over, drizzle on some more olive oil and maple syrup, and roast for about another twenty minutes. I keep an eye on the strips to determine when they're at the perfect softness.

That's how I prefer to eat squash, though I'll eat it any way I can, from delicious grilled zucchini in the spring to butternut squash soup in the winter. Now I turn to the other fruits that are vegetables, or vegetables that are fruits, except for one very strange one, both famous and infamous. Now I turn to the beloved Nightshades.

12.
Solanaceae

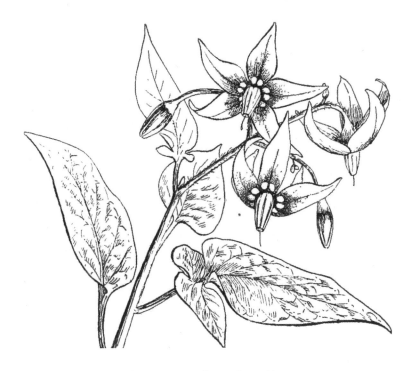

The Nightshades:

Fruit Vegetables Loved by the World's Great Cuisines

I HAD ORIGINALLY PLANNED to put this family at Number One because tomatoes are so fundamental to my farm and my meals—as are peppers—and to the world's greatest cuisines, especially Italian and Latin food. But despite being packed with vitamin C and other key nutrients, the Nightshades, because they are fruits (like the Cucurbits) as opposed to actual vegetables (like the Brassicas and the Chenopods), aren't quite as power packed nutritionally speaking. Another way to look at this eighth family, though, is that I've saved the best—and, in one strange case, perhaps the worst—for last.

Here, we're talking mostly about tomatoes and peppers but also, importantly, about eggplants, tomatillos, and ground cherries, as well as a very strange, infamous vegetable—the "worst" as I just referred to it. These are the Solanaceae, or the Nightshades. I have no idea why they're called the Nightshades, but that's what they're called, so I'll use it as this veggie family's surname.

While I focus mainly on tomatoes and peppers, I'll include one word about green and purple tomatillos, *Physalis philadelphica* and *Physalis ixocarpa*, otherwise known as Mexican husk tomatoes. That word? Underappreciated. There are some great recipes that make use of tomatillos, above and beyond salsa verde. I love them sliced in half, dredged in egg and then corn meal, and fried like green tomatoes or yellow squash but served with a smear of hot pepper jelly. Decadently delicious.

I'll also include a word about the tomatillos' smaller siblings, ground cherries, *Physalis peruviana* and *Physalis pruinosa*, which are like little citrusy cherry tomatoes in a husk. That word? Underappreciated. Ground cherry plants are productive, fast growing, pest free, loved by children, and a great summer snack. Grow some and see what I mean. A volume dedicated to these husk Nightshades, the *Physalis*, is warranted, and maybe I'll write it someday; here, I won't cover them further, as I have a lot to convey about tomatoes, peppers, and the strange one.

RATATOUILLE SORT OF MAKES SENSE. BUT JUST SORT OF.

Peppers are packed with vitamin C. Packed. And they have lots of vitamins A, E, B6, B2 (riboflavin), and B9 (folate), not to mention an array of antioxidants and other types of phytonutrients, like flavonols, flavones, and carotenoids.

While eggplant has some vitamins and minerals and, like peppers, is high in antioxidants, it's not as remarkably a nutritious vegetable. It's food, but not superfood. It is especially healthful, however, when it serves as a meat substitute, replacing the veal in veal Parmesan or the meat in lasagna. My favorite eggplant recipe is meatless meatballs, which, to me, taste better than meatballs with meat. Plus, they're completely free of cholesterol and saturated fat. I usually grow a couple varieties of eggplant, my favorite being the Spanish treasure Listada de Gandia—short and fat with gorgeous purple and white stripes—and the Japanese treasure Ping Tung—long and skinny in glamorous shades of purple.

Similarly, tomatoes are not superfoods, though they do give us the health-promoting phytonutrient lycopene, more of which may be available to our bodies when the tomatoes are cooked. They may be a bit less nutritious overall than peppers, which are also more nutritious when cooked. But we don't eat tomatoes and peppers because they're especially nutritious; we eat them because they're so very delicious.

These three Nightshade fruits are often combined, which goes against the general rule of thumb I've been putting forth of eating across all eight families. But combining peppers and eggplants and tomatoes is not the worst idea nutritionally, as they provide complementary profiles of vitamins, minerals, and phytonutrients despite being closely related. And it's a great idea culinarily, as anyone who eats these fruits roasted or cooked together—meaning anyone who eats ratatouille—well knows. However, combining these vegetables—a delicious choice, as any ratatouille eater can vouch—makes less sense from a nutritional perspective than eating roasted eggplant, turnips, and parsnips; roasted peppers, broccoli, and zucchini; or roasted tomatoes, onions, and carrots, That's because these three roasting options include three families and thus have a much broader nutritional profile. While the ratatouille-style roast gives plenty of vitamins C, A, E, and B6, the pepper, broccoli, and zucchini roast gives not only those same vitamins (thanks to the peppers) but also ample amounts of folate (Vitamin B9), vitamin K, and fiber, along with a broader array of phytonutrients.

Beyond ratatouille, the Nightshades are deliciously combined in countless dishes around the world. Tomatoes and peppers are cherished fruits in nearly every culture. The cuisines of so many Latin American countries, for example, are so extraordinary in large part because of the peppers. Italian food is on the top of many people's lists of favorites in large part because of tomatoes. Like the Alliums and, in many ways, the Umbellifers, the Nightshades make food delicious.

Tomatoes are surely the world's favorite vegetable, for home cooking and for the highest cuisine.

Among the peppers I grow, my favorites are the shishitos (for a pan-seared addiction); pepperoncini (which look similar to shishitos but are the perfect pepper for dipping in veggie dip or, obviously, for pickling); Jimmy Nardello's sweet Italian frying peppers (fried green, like shishitos, or once they turn red and sweeter); petit Marseillais peppers (a beautiful, golden, wavy, thin-walled French heirloom); violet sparkle (because they're shiny and purple—and who doesn't like shiny purple peppers?); poblanos (for delicious stuffed peppers); and both a yellow and a red variety of corno di toro peppers (shaped like a bull's horn and extremely versatile). While the seed catalogs offer a huge variety of peppers, and I'm always tempted to test the latest hybrids, I am very satisfied and happy with, and enthusiastic about, my eight annual pepper favorites. I typically only grow peppers that, like these eight, are low on the Scoville scale, though some years I spice up the farm by adding a few hot pepper plants, which are always so highly productive that I don't know what to do with all the hot little fruits. Those years I make bottled hot sauce, like my "Peaches and Scream" and "Slap Your Farmer."

With countless varieties of sweet and hot peppers available, I no longer grow the most unremarkable of all peppers: bell peppers. It's due to these boring bells that I bring back the grocery store soapbox from which I had railed, profusely and nearly profanely, about iceberg lettuce.

BACK UP ON THE SOAPBOX: BORING BELL PEPPERS

I'll keep it brief: giant green, yellow, and red peppers are strange. They're not strange like the two famous and infamous vegetables that will follow but strange because they're like iceberg lettuce—overappreciated.

Wildly overappreciated. Overused on pizzas when so many delicious heirlooms are available. Overprescribed in countless recipes, primarily because recipe writers can be sure that boring bells will always be on supply in the grocery store. The bell peppers probably have the longest shelf life of all the peppers, especially compared to the more delicate, thin-walled pepper varieties. And it is true that they can be grown to be giant. But it is not true that dishes that call for green, yellow, or red peppers require boring bell peppers. See what the farmers markets have in August and September.

Like iceberg lettuce, I don't grow bell peppers. They're not interesting enough for a vegetable snob like me. They're not tasty enough. We've been bamboozled by the large-scale pepper producers into thinking that bells are the best. But bells are boring because peppers come in such huge variety. It's like relying on the large, perfectly round slicing tomatoes in grocery stores that taste more like unripe green tomatoes. Enough said. I'll step down now.

A STRANGE VEGETABLE THAT BECAME FAMOUS AND THEN INFAMOUS

I previously indicated that we need not concern ourselves with GMO vegetables (at least at the time of this writing), as nearly all our vegetable seeds are either F1 hybrid, open pollinated, or heirloom, that special type of open pollinated. GMOs are primarily concerned with the commodity crops grown for making our underwear; topping off our gasoline tanks; crafting our mayonnaise, ketchup, and countless other ultra-processed foods in the grocery store; and creating cow feed, chicken feed, and pet food; and the like. But there was a time, three decades ago, when the biotech industry took a stab at improving a vegetable above and beyond what Mother Nature could do. And that vegetable was the tomato.

The first GMO plant was produced in the 1980s, and, by 1994, the Flavr Savr tomato was released. Yes, it was called Flavr Savr. The goal was to produce a tomato variety that would hold up better, even when fully ripe, for transporting—a tomato better suited to eighteen-wheelers. Since Mother Nature had not designed tomatoes for long hauls across the country, it would require genetic engineering.

The problem? An enzyme in tomatoes, called polygalacturonase, which can dissolve cell-wall pectin. It was determined to be associated with the natural softening as tomatoes turn from good to bad. That softening, of course, doesn't tolerate a week packed in an eighteen-wheeler very well. Researchers at Calgene, Inc., in Davis, California, strategically inserted a gene that would suppress polygalacturonase accumulation in ripening tomatoes. (Actually, it was two genes; the other allowed the plants to be exposed to a deadly chemical and not die so that the plants that had been successfully genetically modified could be identified. Isn't biotechnology amazing?) A sturdier tomato would ride better and last in grocery store displays longer. Maybe they could even be allowed to ripen on the vine and transported ripe. Thus, the name Flavr Savr. (If you're wondering why anyone would ever harvest an unripe tomato—with no flavor—in the first place, keep reading.)

The USDA approved the Flavr Savr GMO tomato. Then the FDA approved it, with no special labelling necessary. The Flavr Savr tomatoes sold. They were flying off the grocery store displays, red, ripe, and resilient. It would be a new era for big agribusiness tomatoes that could actually be harvested ripe, the only way we would dare to harvest them on a small, local farm.

But, alas, the business ultimately didn't take off, evidently because Calgene was green to tomato harvesting and transport. Calgene had made history but not money. The company was bought by Monsanto in 1997 (for Calgene's technology, not for its not-rotting tomatoes). No more GMO tomatoes, at least for now. Flavr Savr was discontinued.

But back to the issue that Calgene was trying to solve. Let me start by saying that there are two purposes for green tomatoes. One is to fry them like they do down south. The other is to pick them for eighteen-wheelers and then use magic to turn them red for the grocery store. Have you ever had grocery store tomatoes that don't taste much like tomatoes? It's because of the practice of picking green tomatoes and artificially ripening them by ethylene treatment, which gives the ripe tomato color but not the full array of vine-ripened tomato flavors. Ethylene treatment? What?

Well, the basic problem, which Flavr Savr almost fixed before its fall from vegetable grace, is that tomatoes become soft and spoil faster than one can truck them on an eighteen-wheeler from where they are grown (mostly California and Florida) to where northerners like me eat them when they're unavailable here locally, meaning November through June. The best solution to this basic problem would be for northerners like me to not eat tomatoes from November through June (unless canned or otherwise lightly processed, as in marinara sauce made from local tomatoes grown here in the summertime). But people, me included, want their tomatoes. And we want them now—year-round, not just in July through October. When they're grown in California and Florida and sent to grocery stores near me, they have to be picked green so that they remain firm, unbruised, and ready for the long haul. Ethylene gas is used to turn them red.

Ethylene is produced by tomato plants themselves, and some other plants, as part of some fruits' physiology of ripening. Tomatoes exposed to externally applied ethylene (as opposed to ethylene from the plant itself) ripen more uniformly and more quickly; thus, they experience less spoilage than "vine-ripened" tomatoes. But artificially applying ethylene gas to green tomatoes that are too immature just turns them red. Thus, they're pretty much flavorless.

I only pick completely ripe tomatoes on my farm, except for the rare occasions when I have a hankering for fried green tomatoes and don't have tomatillos on hand. And there's no ethylene gas in my barn.

Flavr Savr was famous and then infamous. The big tomato growers ended up having to stick with their green-tomato-and-ethylene-gas practice.

Now on to a famous vegetable that also has become infamous. We haven't seen love-hate like this since broccoli.

A STRANGE VEGETABLE THAT BECAME FAMOUS AND REMAINS FAMOUS (AND INFAMOUS)

Would anyone like french fries with their GMO corn syrup ketchup? It's time for the inevitable story of the strangest of all vegetables covered in our eight chapters—a story that I would rather not tell, but since I resolved to admit frankly and openly to most of my addictions, I must talk about french fries. I, like you, am addicted to them. But I've been working on the habit, and there seems to be at least one effective rule of thumb. Maybe two.

There have been several other vegetables that I deemed too strange for me to grow or to discuss any further, including peanuts (from the Legumes), and artichokes, salsify, and Belgian endive or witloof (all in the Asteraceae family). But this one stands out as quite bizarre, in fact. It's the only one across the sixty or so vegetables within our eight families that is neither a seed, a flower, a leaf, a stem, nor a root. It's a strange plant carbohydrate-storage apparatus called a tuber. And, boy, have we grown to love this tuber.

Meet the potato, *Solanum tuberosum*. I guess that roughly translates from Latin into "the Nightshade that is a tuber." All the other Nightshade vegetables are fruits.

Only a few other vegetables are tubers like potatoes: sweet potatoes (which are in an entirely different family, the Morning Glories, and thus completely unrelated to potatoes); Jerusalem artichokes, or sunchokes (tubers formed by a specific type of perennial sunflower, *Helianthus tuberosus* in the huge Asteraceae family); and some tubers uncommon to many of us that are eaten mostly outside the United

States and which I know very little about, like cassava/yuca, jicama, taro, and yams (actual yams, not sweet potatoes).

Tubers are different from the root vegetables I've covered: the radishes, rutabagas, and turnips among the Brassicas; the onions and shallots among the Alliums, the beets (Chenopods); and the carrots and parsnips (Umbellifers). Root vegetables are roots. There's one per plant, and their function is to draw minerals and moisture from the soil while also storing energy and, importantly, like all other roots, anchoring the plant in the ground. Potatoes are not roots; they are tubers (as in *Solanum tuberosum*).

Tubers—unlike roots, such as carrots—are enlarged storage organs that develop alongside the roots. They're starch storage systems. Few plants have tubers, but for those that do, the starch storage system can help the plant survive a drought, or the winter, and can give the plant enough energy and nutrients to regrow when they are next able. The plant can produce several tubers (unlike radishes, onions, beets, carrots, and the like, which have one root vegetable per plant). And interestingly, unlike root vegetables, which are grown from seeds, you can also use potatoes to create new potato plants (except for when new varieties of potatoes are being created, in which case flowers, cross-pollination, and seeds are involved). That is, you usually grow potatoes by cutting potatoes into quarters or so (actually, there's an art to it, which is sort of fun) and putting those cut pieces of potato into the ground to grow the next crop. You can't do that with a radish or an onion or a beet or a carrot.

Among all the vegetables I've discussed, only the potato is a tuber. That's why I call it strange. It's strange, too, because we've developed a strange fondness for it, unlike *any* other vegetable, a sort of collective addiction. The strange fondness is presumably because a potato is an excellent source of starch, which means calories, which means energy.

Native to beautiful Peru and surrounding countries, now with thousands of varieties, and loved around the world, it's actually pretty tasteless compared to the Nightshade fruits. Unless it's fried. Peoples all around the world eat potatoes and have grown to love french fries and potato chips. Potatoes and the people who love french fries (all of us) made the fast-food companies famous. In turn, the famous fast-food companies now serve us shredded iceberg lettuce and sliced green tomatoes (turned red with ethylene gas). Strangeness breeds strangeness.

Despite thousands of potato varieties, Monsanto evidently felt that a better, patented variety was needed. It created GMO potatoes to, for example, be resistant to the Colorado potato beetle. But when the fast-food and junk food companies—McDonald's, Burger King, Frito-Lay, and the like—decided not to use them due to public pressure, Monsanto kicked its newfangled spud down the road. To the best of my knowledge, most of the potatoes we eat— unlike much of our ketchup (GMO field corn) and much of our mayonnaise (GMO soybeans)—are not GMO potatoes, though GMO potato varieties do exist.

The myriad varieties of potatoes contain water, carbohydrates (primarily starch), a little protein, and negligible fat, along with vitamins B6 and C. They are among the world's top food staples and can be a good source, thankfully, of vodka.

I call potatoes both famous and infamous because, thanks to french fries, chips, tater tots, hash browns, and so on, they are the only vegetable that most people feel they eat *too much of*. No one is worried about their excessive arugula intake or their pea indulgences. And no one stresses about how much Swiss chard they eat or feels guilty over having had too many celery sticks. But most of us feel that we probably eat too many potatoes. That makes this particular vegetable quite strange.

Like everyone else, I eat potatoes, I love potatoes, and, of course, I love fried potatoes like french fries. My own approach to eating potatoes is to do so in moderation, since they have limited nutritional value (compared to the superfood vegetables). I don't view them as bad for you (for example, they have no cholesterol and saturated fat as do animal-based foods like dairy, eggs, and meats), unless they are pushing higher-nutrition foods (like a salad) off your plate. My other potato rule of thumb is that I can eat as many potatoes as I want, even fried, if I grew them myself. Otherwise, I can eat only a few. French fries should come neither fast nor easy.

Despite this all-you-can-eat rule of thumb, I rarely grow potatoes, though my family grew a lot when I was growing up. My main reasons for abstaining are that my farm customers are probably getting sufficient potato intake through other sources, and I don't need to encourage more; they take up a lot of space; and you can never tell what's going on underground. That is, although digging up potatoes is, admittedly, fun, the job might well be met by half of my potatoes having wiry worm holes from wireworms and, as such, being suitable only for the compost pile.

My limited Nightshade space on the farm is dedicated to peppers, eggplants, tomatillos, and ground cherries but most importantly, to tomatoes. Another, somewhat related french fries rule of thumb is that I can eat as much ketchup as I want, no limits, as long as I make my own. It's not hard and, in fact, can be made without corn syrup and without high-fructose corn syrup. But it requires growing extra tomatoes.

LA CASA DEI POMODORI

I've saved the best for last, the best across all these vegetables: delicious heirloom tomatoes and scrumptious cherry and grape tomatoes. I have a close relationship with these fruit vegetables because of the amount of planning involved and the extent of nurturing that goes into their production.

Here on the farm, I grow the ground cherries (tied to trellises), tomatillos (also tied to trellises), eggplants, and peppers out in the open field in full, direct sun, as they all love sunshine and heat, like me and the Cucurbits. Like me, the Nightshades like days, not nights—and sun, not shade. I personally think they should've been called the Sunnydays instead of the Nightshades. Like calling ragweed *Ambrosia*, the Nightshade name seems wrong.

I typically grow six to eight varieties of cherry and grape tomatoes, all different shapes, sizes, and colors. They get blended into pint-size pulp containers that are simply irresistible at the farmers markets. Cherry tomatoes are one of my farm's specialties. I'm addicted to cherry tomatoes, and, to support my habit, I grow a lot of them. I've likely said this about another vegetable, perhaps even dozens of other vegetables, but cherry tomatoes might be my favorite vegetable (fruit) to grow. Among the cherry and grape tomatoes, I have many favorite varieties, though in recent years I've developed a fondness for an F1 hybrid named Valentine. She's delicious, holds up better than most others, does as well in the rain as under the umbrella, and is always perfect.

I usually grow about four to eight varieties of larger, heirloom tomatoes. I prefer those that are not too big (in the three-to-five-ounce range) so that I can include the whole variety in quart-size pulp containers. While there are hundreds to choose from, and I've only tried a small number, my annual favorites are Green Zebra, Japanese Black Trifele, Indigo Apple, and Rose de Berne. Each variety is juicy, sweet, delicious, full of tomato flavor, versatile in the kitchen and in recipes, and striking in appearance. And they're almost completely unavailable in any grocery store.

I started growing tomatoes out in the gardens alongside all the other vegetables across the eight families. I used cages or trellises and let them grow as they wished, without pruning. Yields tended to be less than impressive; disease pressure (like every sort of tomato blight imaginable) was, on the other hand, more than impressive. And, most importantly, summer downpours resulted in major loss of fruit due to cracking and splitting. In fact, growing tomatoes made me dread summer downpours, which a farmer is not supposed to do. The cracking and splitting occur when rapid changes in soil moisture levels (that is, going from fairly dry to being oversaturated from the summer downpour) cause the fruits to expand quicker on the inside—with all that perfectly ripe, juicy tomato flavor—than the tomato skin can grow. Thus, ruptures in the skin. Most of the hundreds of tomato varieties do this, though a few are crack-resistant, like my beloved Valentine grape tomato and my striking Indigo Apple heirloom. Early in my midlife vegetable-growing endeavors, growing tomatoes was not all that satisfying because of the blight diseases and the downpour dilemma.

Then, attending an organic farming conference, I learned about growing tomatoes in "protected culture." It was my first-ever class on growing tomatoes and my first introduction to protected culture. And it changed my life, revolutionizing how I grow tomatoes and intensifying my addiction to cherry tomatoes. During this and several other tomato-growing conference sessions, I heard small-scale organic vegetable farmers repeat what seemed to be a universally accepted mantra: "Once you've grown tomatoes in a hoop house, you'll never grow them in the field again."

It was time for me to build a hoop house.

As you know, I grew up on a dairy farm with a backyard garden, not on a vegetable farm with a backyard milking cow. And having been a doctor all these years, I had never worked on a vegetable farm, much less one with a hoop house. As a big fan of things sturdy, strong, and permanent—like Victory in the middle of the farm—the hoop house I purchased, having done too little research, was indeed sturdy, strong, and permanent. Unlike most hoop houses, it will definitely outlive its builder. The over-sized poles are sunk deep into the ground, each surrounded in concrete. The hoops are extra heavy-duty, intended to withstand not just a downpour but a tornado. The covering is your regular six-mil polyethylene film—umbrella-worthy poly.

It's a small hoop house, for this small farm, at only twenty-four feet wide and thirty-six feet long but more than eleven feet high. I never got around to enclosing the front or the back, and the sides are open up to about four feet. It's literally just a giant umbrella. But rather than "giant umbrella," I refer to it as the Tomato House, or *La Casa dei Pomodori*, in honor of Italy and Italian food.

Outrageously, I packed, across consecutive growing seasons, between 154 and 194 tomato plants into La Casa. They're watered by drip tape on the soil rather than rain, and they're trellised to two leaders with two strings per plant (hanging from cables running along the top of the house) rather than growing as they wish without pruning. And rather than less-than-impressive yields, more-than-impressive disease pressure from every tomato blight imaginable, and major losses from the summer downpours, in La Casa dei Pomodori, yields are great, diseases are nonexistent, and there's never any cracking and splitting. The giant umbrella revolutionized my little tomato operation.

Growing tomatoes, as compared to growing nearly every other vegetable across the eight families, is quite an endeavor. The process starts, of course, during frozen winter months, when it feels like zero outside, and the seed catalogs arrive, tempting late-night curling up by the fireplace with lettuce and tomato porn. I select and order the seeds, and within days they arrive and are logged into my growing notebook. A day or two before March 18, I make my secret-recipe seed-starting mix (mostly peat moss and compost), the same mix that was used in prior weeks for the Brassicas, the Alliums, the Aster Greens, the Umbellifers, and a Chenopod (Swiss chard) and that will be used in about six weeks for the Cucurbit seeds. March 18 is my seed-sowing day for the cherry tomatoes and heirloom tomatoes. Tiny seeds—though not unmanageable like the Aster Greens—one at a time, in seventy-two cells, flat after flat. With daily watering, within a week I'm recording germination rates in my growing notebook.

Within about two weeks, the countless seedlings, about two inches tall, are ready for a larger house, and each gets potted up into four-by-four-inch containers, using the same secret-recipe seed-starting (and seedling) mix. Among our eight families, only the Nightshades (and the fussy celery) on my little farm get potted up. And they all get potted up: tomatoes, peppers, eggplants, tomatillos, and ground cherries. It's a lot of potting, days on end. The pretty, perky, fast-growing tomato plants stay in their pots in the greenhouse for another five weeks, until about May 8.

May 8 or thereabouts, depending on the ten-day forecast and once fully assured that there will not be another frost, is tomato-planting day. By this time, the plants are ten to twenty inches tall and very ready to move from their square pots into a much larger house, La Casa dei Pomodori. They're not supposed to be planted this close, but on my compact farm, I must plant everything too close, so I plant them about nine inches apart. As soon as they're planted, they get their first trellis string, hung from the top of the hoop house and attached to each plant's main leader (the top of the plant that is growing). They grow quickly. Within a couple of weeks, each gets a second string, attached to their second most robust leader. We then strive to keep them pruned, snipping away all the other growing tips (suckers), so that each plant is two long vines, heading toward the top of the hoop house, repeatedly clipped to the trellis strings every few feet. The race is on to see which variety gets there first, up to eleven feet tall. Black Cherry, one of the heirloom cherry tomatoes, usually wins.

By the middle of July, the cherry tomatoes are arriving, in all of their shapes, sizes, and colors. Green Zebra and the other heirloom slicers are just a couple weeks behind. Summer has arrived, my body is fully energized, my mind at its sharpest, my hopes at their highest, my plate at its healthiest.

Now, with these delicious fruits, I am eating well, just how the Delamaters ate well, in July, August, and September. In the summer, I have no thoughts of the long, cold, dark winter months of planning and physical and psychological hibernation that will eventually arrive, though the Delamaters undoubtedly not just thought ahead toward those months but seriously planned for them.

BLISTERED SHISHITO PEPPERS, CHERRY TOMATO CAPRESE SALAD

In late summer, I eat a lot of peppers, especially fried Jimmy Nardello's (prepared just like the shishito recipe given below, except halved since they're larger), stuffed poblano peppers, and stuffed sweet peppers. Shishitos have become trendy in restaurants in recent years, whether as an appetizer or a tapas small plate, and they're very easy to make at home.

My Blistered Shishito Peppers. I sell shishito peppers in pint pulp containers at the farmers markets. They can occasionally be found in bags in the grocery store, though inevitably not as local and thus not as fresh. The ideal size, based on my palate and a lot of experience with growing shishitos, is about the size of your index finger. Any smaller and they tend to become flaccid; any larger and they're less pleasurable to eat whole (with too-large seeds and too-thick skins). Like so many of my other farm-to-table recipes, I start with a large skillet and a couple of tablespoons of olive oil. Once it's hot on the stove at medium heat, I throw in the whole pint (or bag) of shishitos and toss them so that they're all lightly coated with olive oil. I let them cook until they just begin to turn golden brown and blister on one side, then toss again. Repeat. On the third or so repeat, so that all sides are blistered, I sprinkle them with just enough sea salt to make them addictive. Then, they're done and ready to be eaten, whole, by picking them up by the stem, biting off the pepper, and discarding the stem.

Blistered shishitos are a great way to start a meal. Most are mild and delicious, but one hopes that about one in twenty will have some unexpected fire. The next course, a caprese salad before a light, simple pasta entrée, makes use of the never-ending supply of summertime cherry and grape tomatoes.

My Cherry Tomato Caprese Salad. When the tomatoes are ripe, I eat as many as I can, knowing that wintertime tomatoes from the grocery store are going to be less than satisfying. When the basil is ripe in early to mid-summer, I eat a caprese salad nearly every day, altering the ingredients and looks each time. My favorite is to simply take a pint of cherry tomatoes (ideally of all different colors and shapes) and cut each one in half. I drizzle some extra virgin olive oil on them and salt them. I lay them out on a salad plate, add chunks of fresh (ideally local) mozzarella cheese, and plenty of coarsely cut or gently torn Italian basil. I again toss it gently and then drizzle the salad with balsamic vinegar, or, for a sweeter version if I just had shishito peppers, balsamic glaze. I've never had a dinner guest who didn't find it heavenly.

13.

How I Eat, and Why

MY SIMPLE RULE OF THUMB FOR HEALTHY EATING, which I refer to as *eight on my plate*, is a whole-foods, plant-predominant eating pattern with a broad array of vegetables from these eight families of plants. Eating this way requires getting veggie smarts and learning about the eight families, which I've done, and which I hope that many others will do. It might come natural to many gardeners and small farmers, but most eaters—despite knowing how spaghetti and penne pasta, and beef tenderloin and pork loin, are and are not related—often do not know the relationships between beets and carrots or arugula and radishes. The beetles and the groundhogs definitely know those relationships, and I think that if we do as well, then we can select what to eat in a way that will optimize both our physical health and our mental health.

A PESCETARIAN PRESBYTERIAN

I've come to embrace a whole-foods, plant-predominant eating pattern for at least eight reasons.

First, with such a passion for plants, with green thumbs, and with my specific veggie addictions, I want more room on my plate for vegetables. Things that aren't as delicious to me, like meats and breads, are thus crowded out by the vegetables I savor.

Second, I believe in the many benefits of growing my own food. It brings about great satisfaction. I like growing vegetables and fruits; I'm not interested in growing pigs, cows, or grains. Thus, I prefer to eat vegetables.

Third, I really enjoy making my own food in my own kitchen, especially with vegetables just picked from the gardens. This allows me to focus on whole foods and to minimize ultra-processed foods.

Fourth, a couple of health indicators, like creeping cholesterol levels, suggested that I would benefit from a whole-foods, plant-predominant eating pattern. To the extent that my creeping cholesterol was from dietary sources (and roughly 25 percent probably was), it was worth recalling from medical school that cholesterol is found exclusively in animal foods (meat, eggs, dairy, cheese, and so on); vegetables, fruits, grains, and other plant foods contain none.

Fifth, I became board certified in lifestyle medicine, and in my studies, the science behind the health benefits of this way of eating were undeniable. For example, both soluble and insoluble fiber are important for normalizing bowel movements, maintaining bowel and microbiome health, and lowering risk of colorectal cancer; lowering cholesterol levels; helping to control blood sugar levels; and lowering risk of heart disease, prediabetes, and type 2 diabetes. Fiber is found exclusively in plant foods, completely absent in animal foods.

Sixth, I read about concentrated animal feeding operations (CAFOs) and watched documentaries about them and related topics. It's not how we should feed and care for animals, and it's not how we should eat meat. On the other hand, I'm not opposed to eating local meat.

Seventh, I read about and watched documentaries on ultra-processed foods, the massive industrial food complex, and the politics involved. The situation we're in is dire—not one for pondering, not one needing more research, but a mess that necessitates change right now. Granny Hannah never had a single bite of ultra-processed food, ate well, and lived to be seventy-seven despite having been born in 1790. Yes, seventy-seven. My Granny Essie Mae, having lived to eighty-five, rarely ate ultra-processed food, except in the later decades of her life when it was becoming ever more ubiquitous and touted for its convenience. It is very hard not to eat ultra-processed food nowadays, at nearly every meal, given our food environment. But we don't have to. Avoiding it just requires substantial effort and commitment.

Eighth, life is already too short—why would I eat in a way that is bound to make it shorter?

For me, embracing a whole-foods, plant-predominant eating pattern does not mean I'm a vegan (though perhaps I will be someday); nor does it mean I'm a strict vegetarian. I'm a flexitarian at times (such as when I eat local meat), a pescetarian for many of my dinners, and a presbyterian on some of my Sundays after eating quiche and salad. Just kidding. For me, a whole-foods, plant-predominant eating pattern means I try to eat smart, and the key to eating smart is eating food replete with diverse vegetables. It's not hard to do so now that I have veggie smarts.

HOMEMADE QUICHE AND SALAD, HOLD THE HOME FRIES AND BACON

I'll leave lunch as an open question—as it's easily figured out using the eight-on-my-plate approach to deciding what to eat—but I'll say a few words about what I eat for breakfast and then what I like for dinner. First, breakfast.

Breakfast is the strangest of the three meals to me, as we have settled on a very restricted menu, at least from the perspective of my European, and British in particular, heritage. Breakfast is about grains in the form of toast, breads, biscuits, muffins, bagels, pancakes, waffles, doughnuts, oatmeal, and cereals eaten with milk. Breakfast is also about eggs, lots of eggs, and dairy, including cottage cheese, yogurt, and the milk that we eat cereals with. And breakfast is about meats—bacon, ham, and sausage, in particular. To some extent, breakfast may also be about fruit, but usually only the fruits that are sweet. Of course, we like to include fried potatoes, like home fries and hash browns, which is unsurprising since we like fried potatoes at any meal, if not at every meal.

That's basically what breakfast is about: grains; eggs; dairy; meats like bacon, ham, and sausage; maybe fruit; and hopefully some fried potatoes. It's probably pretty clear where I'm going with this.

Where are the vegetables at breakfast? Why don't we eat vegetables before noon? What's going on with this strange meal that starts our day? I haven't done the research to figure it out, and maybe an explanation already exists. Is it just cultural? Familial and societal traditions? Or is there some strange physiological underpinning? Does it have something to do with the fact that we've been asleep for so long? Or that we've been deprived of calories during all those hours of sleep? I'm sure that others have asked and answered these questions. I personally find breakfast to be the strangest of the three meals because it almost entirely excludes vegetables. But with my approach to eating—eight on my plate—even at breakfast the goal is to eat some vegetables alongside all those other delicious creations. Or in lieu of them.

I'm not opposed to eating grain-things for breakfast, or to eating eggs. My farm did, after all, embark upon the stuck-at-home pandemic venture of laying hens, and they give us a lot of very fresh eggs. They're dropped by the hens at five AM and in my frying pan by seven. And I'm not opposed to dairy. I did, after all, grow up on a dairy farm, drinking a lot of raw milk, and I seem to have turned out just fine. In fact, I attribute (or misattribute) all that raw milk to making me smart, strong, and studly. While I'm not opposed to eggs and dairy (though they seem strange things to eat and drink if you really stop and think about it), for some people, probably most people, the saturated fat and cholesterol in eggs and dairy warrant placing limits and making substitutions. I also have to say—not as a farmer but as a doctor interested in preventing and reversing disease—that the bacon, ham, and sausage are just bad. Everyone knows that, so my recommendation is not radical: we should stop eating it. At least how it's currently produced and eaten.

My point is that I personally would like to eat some vegetables with breakfast. My distant British relatives who stayed in the homeland do in fact eat some vegetables at breakfast, as a "full English breakfast" includes grilled tomatoes and baked beans (alongside all the cereal, toast, eggs, bacon, ham, and sausage). I've always thought—perhaps it's genetic—that tomatoes and beans seem to me perfect for breakfast. But with eight on my plate, I want to get in a few other vegetables. I probably won't get eight families in, but a couple would be good, three even better, and anything beyond that undoubtedly healthy compared to the delicious mainstays that usually make up our breakfast.

For me, with all this produce and with dinners that inevitably are too sizeable to eat in one sitting, breakfast is often about leftovers, like leftover sides without an entrée, or even leftover pizza. Yes, a grown man—a doctor and a farmer—eats leftover pizza for breakfast. I'll tell you about my pizza. Eating delicious leftovers serves the dual purpose of getting some vegetables for breakfast and not wasting perfectly good, healthy food. Aside from leftovers, for me, there is one perfect breakfast fare that functions as a delicious vegetable-delivery meal: quiche.

I used to think that quiche was fancy, only for fancy restaurants. Now, I think it's the perfect breakfast in the spring, summer, and fall when fresh vegetables abound. And somehow it just calls for a side salad next to it on the plate. Frittatas come in close behind it, with omelets, for me, a distant third.

Quiche is very easy to make (pie crust, vegetables, eggs and milk, and a little cheese—but the key is lots of vegetables), and it keeps well in the refrigerator for several days. When I make quiche, I first think of what vegetables I have on hand, preferably freshly picked from the gardens that morning. Then I consider what would taste good together when combined. Then I think about eight on my plate, and if there is a way to optimize the vegetable content that this vegetable-delivery meal is going to provide. What's available? What would taste good? What will be most nutritious?

I've abandoned making the overly restrictive customary quiches like quiche Lorraine (bacon or ham and eggs), quiche au fromage (cheese and eggs), or even quiche Florentine (as I'm going for more vegetables than just spinach, and that's coming from someone addicted to spinach despite being a complete failure at growing spinach). Quiche gives us a chance to savor vegetables in the form of a delicious vegetable pie. Who wouldn't want pie for breakfast? I admittedly cheat and use the rolled-up pie crusts in a box found in the refrigerated section of the grocery store, though one of my culinary goals next year is to learn to make my own pie crusts. Here are two of my favorite quiches incorporating the families that I have now learned well, starting with a Brassica, accompanied by an Allium, and so on.

My Green Quiche. Chopped broccoli from the farm plus thinly sliced leeks from the farm plus a handful of frozen English baby peas—which I don't grow, so straight from the bag in the freezer—plus washed and chopped spinach, embarrassingly, from the grocery store. I call it my green quiche—four shades of green. If I serve it alongside a delicate salad of sweet heirloom lettuce with sliced cucumber and a small, sliced heirloom tomato, all from the farm, I've just served myself, or others, seven families of vegetables. Not to worry, I can eat some celeriac purée tonight with dinner. Eight families today. This quiche-and-salad breakfast is so filling that I need no home fries or hash browns, nor do I need toast.

My Autumn Quiche. Here's another one: a thinly sliced small storage onion from the farm plus chopped Swiss chard from the farm plus a handful of chopped radicchio from the farm plus bite-sized chunks of butternut squash from the farm, roasted last night for dinner. Yes, radicchio and butternut squash in quiche. If I serve it alongside a small salad of arugula with sliced cherry tomatoes, both from the farm, I've just created a breakfast pie with six families of vegetables. I can eat some celery sticks with hummus for lunch. Eight families today. That's obviously very healthy.

To be even healthier, quiche can be made crustless (and frittatas have no crust anyway), and some of the eggs can be replaced with egg whites. Quiche, of course, is not the only way to have vegetables at breakfast, but it's a delicious and easy vegetable-delivery meal. Once I practiced making it a few times, I never needed a recipe again.

HOMEMADE PIZZA AND SALAD, HOLD THE CARDBOARD AND PLASTIC

I have four thoughts to share about how I most prefer to eat dinner. Actually, I have lots of thoughts about eating dinner, including what I'm going to eat tonight in this old stone house after drafting this next-to-last chapter. But I'm going to limit myself to four.

My first thought about dinner is that entrées are overappreciated, and dinners without entrées are underappreciated.

Not every dinner needs to have an entrée. Having an entrée usually means meat of some sort, and if a meat can be pushed off the plate to make room for vegetables, the meal will always be healthier. Some of my favorite dinners, whether at home or in restaurants, are ones with four vegetable "sides." Four vegetable sides always create a square meal. A delicious, square, four-sided meal might be collard greens plus pinto beans with diced onions plus fried yellow squash plus spinach salad, lightly dressed, with finely sliced celery and a few sliced ground cherries. The counting is easy by now: that adds up to seven families. No entrée needed. I can eat some lettuce or radicchio tomorrow.

Another square, four-sided meal might be roasted broccoli rabe with onions plus white beans and escarole plus honey roasted carrots plus tomato and cucumber salad. Seven families. No entrée needed. There will be Swiss chard on the farm for tomorrow. I love savoring sides and only sides. Four sides. Always square.

My second thought about dinner? Dinners don't have to be four-sided to be square. I like having two main dishes that balance one another well, like roasted root vegetables and a salad. For the roots, I could do turnips plus onions plus beets plus carrots plus potatoes. For the salad, I could have a sweet heirloom lettuce with chickpeas. Seven families. No entrée needed. I'll have some cantaloupe with my quiche at breakfast.

Another among the myriad two-part dinners is an Asian stir-fry served with a side of homemade kimchi. My spring kimchi has napa cabbage, radishes, and carrots. That as a side to the stir-fry—let's say scallions, snow peas, yellow squash, sliced shishito peppers, and celery—gives us seven families. I don't have any spinach on the farm in the spring (or in any other season, embarrassingly), but there will be Swiss chard for tomorrow.

My third thought about eating dinner pertains to eating dinner out. When ordering, I think about eating vegetables from across eight families as a way to optimize the taste and the healthfulness of the meal. One of my favorite Chinese meals is to simply order "mixed vegetables in black bean sauce." It usually comes with broccoli and napa cabbage (from the Brassicas), onions (the Alliums), green beans and snow peas (the Legumes, same as the black beans), carrots and celery (the Umbellifers), and zucchini (the Cucurbits). That's five families in one entrée. Or at an Indian restaurant, rather than just the paneer cheese and lentil curry (which is delicious), I'm more likely to go for the mixed vegetable dish that includes cauliflower, onions, chickpeas and green peas, carrots, yellow squash, and potatoes. Six families.

Finally, my fourth thought about dinner is, in one word, pizza. Yes, I'm a doctor, and, yes, I'm trying to eat more pizza for my health.

Like quiche for breakfast, pizza for dinner is a great vegetable-delivery meal, especially when served, like quiche, with a salad. We're talking homemade pizza (as delivered pizza is usually unhealthy), heavy on the vegetables. I'm also a believer in eating more pasta—again, yes, I said eating more (not less) pasta—following the same two caveats (a homemade dish, heavy on the vegetables).

For my pizza at home, I prefer thin crust, and I like using whatever is available on the farm—seasonal pizza. Thin crust plus tomato sauce plus chopped kale plus summer onions plus petit Marseillais, Jimmy Nardello's, or another non–bell pepper plus diced zucchini. Served with a lettuce and pea shoot salad, that's six families.

The eight-on-my-plate approach, when using seasonal, local vegetables and made at home, is not just exceptionally good for our physical health and our mental health; it's good for our land and our environment. It creates a minimal carbon footprint from the transporting of vegetables and other ingredients; there's no need for cardboard, like the pizza boxes that used to be trees; and we can minimize single-use plastics like kitchen-to-landfill take-out containers, or even plastics that are recycled.

EIGHT ON MY PLATE FOR MY PHYSICAL HEALTH

It's probably obvious by now that eating many vegetables from eight different families of plants is good for your body. Eating this way gives us all the carbohydrates and protein we need, along with healthy fats rather than unhealthy ones.

I've said in discussing the Legumes that the protein's in the beans. But it's actually in most of our vegetables. We eat protein for the amino acids so that we can build our own proteins. Think about the big, muscular black angus cows in the pasture, eating grass and broadleaf plants/weeds all day and making massive amounts of protein, as complete vegetarians—vegans, in fact. Although beans are packed with protein, many vegetables have substantial protein content. While most are incomplete in the protein arena in that they don't have all the amino acids we need to build all our own proteins, the solution is simple—don't eat just one plant food; eat a variety of them.

Yes, most vegetables contain a good amount of protein, and if we eat diverse vegetables and mix legumes with grains, we will get all the amino acids we need, despite having been bamboozled into the idea that we need to eat animal-derived foods (dairy, eggs, and meats) to get the protein we need. It's all been a matter of lobbying and marketing. Vegetables, from adzuki beans to watercress, give us all the protein we need with fewer calories than dairy, eggs, and meats. Plus, dairy, eggs, and meats have no health-promoting, disease-fighting fiber. Zero. Zilch. Even if you eat the eggshells and the bones.

Eating diverse vegetables across eight families gives us an abundance of fiber needed for health. It also gives us a full array of micronutrients—vitamins and minerals. All these plants also give us phytonutrients, plant compounds that serve a nutritional and biochemical purpose, with antioxidant, inflammation-reducing, neuroprotective, and cancer-reducing properties. Anthocyanins are in red and purple vegetables and fruits, carotenoids in dark orange, yellow, and green ones. Flavonoids. Indoles. Lutein. Lycopene in tomatoes. And the list goes on.

In all these ways—the right carbohydrates, the right proteins, the right fats, an abundance of fiber, a full array of vitamins and minerals, and the bounty of compounds that only plants provide—eight on my plate is undoubtedly good for my health. It's about being smart with vegetables. I believe it will improve my overall health profile, reduce my risk for many or most diseases, help reduce the impact of any diseases I will develop, and allow me to live a longer life. This eight-on-my-plate approach is good for my heart, good for my gastrointestinal system, good for my liver, good for my kidneys, good for my eyes, and good for my skin. It's a way of eating, or a way of striving to eat, healthy—not a diet.

EIGHT ON MY PLATE FOR MY MENTAL HEALTH

What's good for the gut, the kidneys, and the skin, is good for the brain. The fact that eight on my plate is good for the brain should come as no surprise—our brains are organs like the others, though unfathomably complex and obviously exceedingly precious. We should care for it. Like our other parts, it deserves our eating a great diversity of vegetables from eight different families of plants.

I had thought to go on a tangent here about the emerging and compelling science on food and mood, how to eat to beat some of the most common mental illnesses, nutritional psychiatry, the connection between the gut and the mind, diets for happiness, and the like. But others have written on these topics with great aptitude. Suffice it to say that the brain benefits from the macronutrients, micronutrients, and phytonutrients that plants provide.

What I will say, though, is that eating well—that is, eight on my plate—makes me feel better. I have more energy, crisper thinking, higher aspirations, more adrenaline, more productive exercising, and more restorative sleep. But perhaps most importantly, with my newfound veggie smarts, I feel a sense of achievement—accomplishment, actually—in having done what I know is good for my health, for my life, and even for our land and our environment.

I should say that I experience that sense of accomplishment "at times," not always. If I've suggested that eight on my plate is how I actually eat, I have likely exaggerated my success. This simple premise is how I *strive* to eat. It's my goal, many days accomplished, some days not. You don't have to be perfect to be a success.

As a mental health professional and a lifestyle medicine expert, I try to help people move beyond their addictions. But as I've described, somewhat (but only somewhat) jokingly, I'm addicted to several vegetables, which are addictions that I have no need to move beyond. My currently identified addictions cross five of the eight families: arugula, snow peas, spinach, fried yellow squash, roasted winter squash, blistered shishitos, cherry tomatoes, and, of course, french fries (not potatoes, but french fries). This latter drug of choice is the only one that I am trying to work on. Group therapy is likely warranted, as I'm not the only one with the problem. As I've described, I have some special rules of thumb for french fries: moderation, avoiding plate takeover so that there's room for salad, and eating as many potatoes as I want, even fried, if I grew them myself. Similarly, I can eat as much ketchup as I want, with no concern about GMO high-fructose corn syrup, if I make my own ketchup. It only requires fresh, ripe tomatoes, apple cider vinegar, brown sugar, salt, and some seasoning, like cinnamon, garlic powder, and onion powder.

I know my vegetable addictions and hope to acquire others, and I encourage you to know and nurture yours. I have yet to develop an addiction among the Alliums, though I use them so frequently when cooking other vegetables that it might appear to be one. I'm also not yet addicted to the Aster

Greens, mainly because openly acknowledging an addiction to lettuce just sounds too strange. That said, I am so fascinated by the chicories of the Aster Greens that I plan to write a farmer-nerd book or blog series about them, so that's pretty intense, perhaps bordering on addiction. And, finally, I am not yet addicted to the Umbellifers, though honey roasted carrots are so close to ambrosia that it would not be unimaginable. Same for parsley-walnut pesto. Repeating some dishes leads to habits, which lead to cravings.

Silliness aside, this addiction narrative is just to suggest that I have developed a close and fun, if not funny, relationship with vegetables, and I think that my mental health is better off for having done so. The growing led to the craving, and the craving meant needing more room on my plate for the craved-for foods. That meant less room for meats and breads, which I no longer crave.

EATING VEGGIES FROM OTHER FAMILIES, AND SEEDS AND NUTS

I don't know why, among more than four hundred families of flowering plants with more than ten thousand genera and about three hundred thousand species, nearly all our vegetables come from just a few genera and species within just eight families. I assume that it has something to do with humans having tasted many thousands of plants and settling on a manageable few tasty ones to focus on as food-worthy and thus cultivation-worthy. In recent times, selection of specific varieties has gone in two directions: increased diversity and decreased diversity.

Increased? Intentional, controlled crossbreeding (or cross-fertilizing or cross-pollinating) has resulted in many new hybrid cultivars grown from F1 hybrid seeds. Great new carrots, celery, radicchio, peppers, tomatoes, and so on. Decreased? At the same time, many open-pollinated and heirloom varieties that are less suitable to large-scale growing, harvesting, and transporting have become difficult to find. Only small farms and home gardeners are growing them. Although our remote ancestors' tasting of plants resulted in culinary and nutritional reasons for the few plant species that we eat, production and supply-chain reasons have shaped the particular cultivars available to eat today.

I've chosen to focus on eight families because all the vegetables on my farm come from these eight, as do the vast majority of all of our vegetables. Yet there are a few vegetables from other families that are one-hit wonders. These include asparagus from the Asparagaceae family; okra from the Malvaceae family, which also includes cotton; sweet potatoes from the Morning Glory family, Convolvulaceae; and mâche, or corn salad, or lamb's lettuce, a delicious little salad leaf from the Honeysuckle family, Caprifoliaceae. One-hit wonders, but delicious.

Other vegetables that I've neglected, from among many, simply because I have not grown them, include chayote (from the Cucurbits, but in a different genus than the three that I covered), fiddleheads (from ferns, not flowering plants), ginger, nasturtium, purslane, rhubarb, sorrel, water chestnuts, and yucca (the latter in the Asparagaceae family along with asparagus), as well as the others given in "A Glossary for Getting Smart About Veggies" at the beginning of the book. Of course, there are others eaten and savored outside of the

American experience. And, of course, there are all the delicious mushrooms, which aren't plants but fungi.

Had I covered herbs, aside from the leaves and seeds of the Umbellifer Herbs (angelica, caraway, chervil, cilantro, dill, fennel, parsley, and others), I would have needed to pay tribute to the Lamiaceae (or Labiatae) family, the mint and sage family, which includes basil, lavender, lemon balm, marjoram, mint, oregano, rosemary, sage, thyme, and a number of others. They make so many of our vegetables taste so good.

Perhaps the most important family, around the globe, in terms of staple foods (setting aside potatoes), is the Poaceae, or Gramineae: flowering plants that are monocots like the Alliums and with which we are all to some extent familiar, as the family supplies not just food but most of our outdoor carpet. The Poaceae, or the Grasses, give us barley, corn (which is a particularly strange grass, especially if you read about the silks and how they work), millet, oats, rice, rye, wheat, ancient farro wheats like einkorn, and others, including sugarcane, sorghum, lemongrass, and bamboo. This family feeds us around the world; feeds our meat-, milk-, and egg-producing animals; gives us the needed ingredients for our much-needed beer, rum, vodka, and whisky; and helps to fuel our cars. An entire volume could be dedicated to the Grasses.

Finally, I've spoken too little about the importance of eating seeds and nuts. These tiny powerhouses of nutrition—like pepitas or pumpkin seeds, sunflower seeds, chia seeds, flaxseeds, sesame seeds, almonds, Brazil nuts, cashews, hazelnuts, macadamia nuts, pecans, pistachios, walnuts, and others—offer a myriad of health benefits. Like all the dry beans or "pulses" within the Legumes, packed with protein, healthy fats, many micronutrients, and a rich fiber content, seeds and nuts support overall health and aid digestion while promoting a healthy digestive system. Additionally, the array of antioxidants found in seeds and nuts can help combat oxidative stress, supporting heart health and potentially lowering the risk of chronic diseases like cardiovascular disease and type 2 diabetes. With their versatility, seeds and nuts can easily be added to meals (like sunflower seeds sprinkled on almost any homemade salad) or enjoyed as a snack, making it convenient to reap their nutritional rewards and contribute to a balanced way of eating. I make my own trail mix combining as many of these nuts and seeds as possible (along with some raisins, dried cranberries, and, of course, mini dark chocolate chips) and eat a handful each day.

A NATURAL-BORN BERRY PICKER

Because I've been writing about vegetables rather than fruits (except for the Cucurbits and the Nightshades, which give us fruits that we call vegetables, or vegetables that are horticulturally fruits), I haven't mentioned the Rosaceae, or Rose family, which, in addition to roses, gives us strawberries, raspberries, blackberries, almonds, apples, apricots, cherries, peaches, pears, plums, and others. A story about eating sweet fruits, instead of about eating vegetables from across eight families, would have had the Rosaceae as the centerpiece. Such a story would also have covered the Ribes (currants), which is the only genus in the Grossulariaceae family, in a way that would have been more detailed than my tribute to

Granny's red currant bush and all the ones I grow with her and my green thumbs.

Although growing and eating these fruits would need to be covered in a different volume, I like eating fruits as much as I like eating vegetables. My general rule of thumb is that it's alright to partake of exotic fruits from the grocery store (bananas, mangoes, oranges, pineapples, and the like) on occasion (but only on occasion, given their travel distances), but I can eat as many Ulster County apples as I want, year-round. Apple sauce, apple butter, apple pie. There are a lot of apples in my area, along with some peaches, pears, and plums.

I'm not much for growing fruit trees, but I was born to grow other fruits as I was born to grow vegetables, with strawberries, currants, black raspberries, blackberries, and blueberries at the top of the list. It must be a genetic thing. I like growing them, and I like picking them. You're either a natural-born berry picker, or you're not. Are you? Or do you not know?

When I see a berry bush loaded with ripe berries, I must pick them. I'm magnetically drawn to them, and both hands start moving synchronously. One from berry to bucket, the other from berry to mouth. Currants on the farm, wild raspberries along the roadsides, wild blueberries in the woods—it doesn't matter. I've stopped my taxi driver before, twice, in two different cities, en route from the airport to downtown, on a busy highway, at the sighting of ripe wild raspberries in the edge of the woods. Both times, the drivers were reluctant to pull over and back up when I blurted out the need to stop, but they did upon my atypical, boisterous proclamation of being a berry expert (more convincing than just being a natural-born berry picker). Both times, meter running, I told them, "Wait here for just a couple of minutes. It'll be worth it." I'm sure that the truckers and drivers zooming by assumed I was stepping into the woods for other reasons. Both times, the cab drivers were delighted with the unusually sweet berries. I don't think either was a natural-born berry picker, so they were most grateful that I am.

I'm a natural-born berry picker, meaning that I'm good at picking berries—efficiently using both hands, nimbly plucking the fully ripe ones, leaving those not quite ready for a later day. Unfortunately, most people *don't know* if they're a natural-born berry picker because they haven't had the opportunity to make the determination. But I think that everyone should figure it out, one way or the other. Those who determine that they are will feel a calling to grow their own berries; the calling isn't really resistible, be it on an under-an-acre farm, in a raised bed for June strawberries, or in a simple planter on the balcony overlooking the cityscape. But the calling is only realized if one comes to find out, perhaps in the woods, if they are, in fact, a natural-born berry picker. For those who discover that they are not, they will likely become much more appreciative of the natural-born berry pickers of the world and will be grateful for the berries that we have picked for them.

I'm sure that some of the Delamaters kids raised, or born and raised, in this old stone house were natural-born berry pickers. Those who weren't undoubtedly really appreciated their siblings who were.

14.

Eating for Health,
Eating Sustainably

GROWING UP, spending long summer days outdoors in the cow pastures and in the vegetable gardens, ours and Granny's, surrounded by siblings, cousins, aunts and uncles, and their gardens, I figured that I would always grow my own vegetables for the summer, with frozen and canned ones for the winter. I didn't know to think otherwise. I never figured, though, that I would someday live in an old stone house that would prove to be as old as any history lesson taught in school. And I never figured that I would become a vegetable farmer growing vegetables for others.

After a long hiatus from the gardens, in the back and in front of classrooms and lecture halls—a hiatus of some quarter century—a little garage-sized garden beside a garage in the Hudson Valley, a place I had previously never heard of, found me. That garden called me to grow. I filled the garden with plants that would give vegetables that filled my kitchen, and I then had sod turned to soil to build a little under-an-acre organic vegetable farm. It fed a lot of people.

Amid the painstaking, inner-deliberating seed selection in the cold, frozen months, I was also called, by this old stone house, to learn who lived here before me so that I could grow a deep respect for them. All those families, with grannies from Hannah to Yancey, came to feel like my own families, their gardens undoubtedly planted with the same aspirations, passions, and green thumbs as mine. My gardens, expanding each year into a little farm, taught me about other families—eight families of plants and the cousins and siblings within them, these generous plants, dear friends who have given me guidance and nurturance. I now eat healthier because of this journey.

HOW HANNAH, CORNELIUS, AND THE KIDS ATE

By the summer of 1830, the Delamater family had settled into their new stone house dated 1828. With nine mouths to feed, they would need to have a bountiful summer—bountiful enough not just for summer but for the entire fall and winter, and even through early spring.

The family grew nearly all their food. They never went to a restaurant. There was no takeout or delivery. There were no supermarkets. All their meals were homegrown and homemade. For Hannah, needing to quickly recover after each birth (and perhaps her whole-foods way of eating helped in that recovery), the gardens and cooking consumed most of her time and energy, with any of the girls old enough to help taking part.

Hiram and Jonathan worked with the cows, sheep, and pigs, Sally and Rosaland with the chickens. Hannah tended to the raspberries, and at least one of the kids, if not half of them, were undoubtedly natural-born berry pickers like her and me. Cornelius stacked stone walls, built fences and hedgerows, and planned the planting, tending, harvesting, and storing of the crops, all tasks that I share with him here on his land, my land, our land—not really our land.

For the few food items the family did not produce, good relationships with neighbors along the long winding road toward the Church at Klyne Esopus were key: bartering excess bushels of winter squash for sacks of flour, cabbage for apples, beets and carrots for asparagus crowns for a newly prepared garden. And they undoubtedly traded seeds.

The family did not have a detached kitchen in a building separate from the house, which, if they had, would have kept the house cleaner, cooler, and fresher. It would have required building yet another stone structure, a project the growing family could not afford. Hannah and the girls cooked instead here at a hearth that many years since was converted to a much smaller coal-burning, and then wood-burning, fireplace in our dining room. They sometimes used an open flame, but often they cooked with hot coals underneath a Dutch oven standing on three legs, not unlike Granny's iron apple butter kettle that sits right next to my garden beside the garage.

Obviously, there was no electricity, and so no toasters or microwaves. No glass bottles of salad dressing, and no purchased or ultra-processed food of any sort. In fact, there was no glass in the kitchen, just wood containers and some pewter items. No countertops. No fans. No colanders. No napkins. No cookbooks. Things were pretty basic.

Eggs from the family's ten or so hens were collected daily by the girls, probably in a way that looks almost exactly like how I collect the eggs each day from our fifteen. In their case, though, once hens stopped producing, they, and most of the roosters along the way, would be roasted outside in the summer or boiled inside in the winter.

Milk was brought in from the family's one or two cows daily, probably by the boys, the cream allowed to rise to the top and then going into the butter churn. Like eggs, both milk and butter were always on hand. Meats, primarily pork, were cured by smoking, drying, brining, and salting, all drawing moisture out of the meat to prevent spoiling. These skills are long forgotten among homeowners today, even those in the countryside. Knowledge lost.

Any vegetables that could be cured for the long winter, or that could remain cool by being "put down" in the root cellar for several months, would be planted heavily each summer and fall. In addition to milk, eggs, bread, butter, and meats, November, December, and January meals would rely heavily on cabbage, turnips, onions, beets, carrots, and potatoes. February and March would see few vegetables at the table, except those that were pickled, along with the winter squash and dry beans that would last until young greens and roots were again available in April and May.

March and April were about a gradual reawakening, rejuvenation, resurrection. May and June were the most glorious months; July, August, and September the most bountiful—for the Delamaters and for me.

Rather than the winter months being ones of intense planning, as they are for me, the summer months were the planning ones for them, needing as they did to ensure enough vegetables were grown, cured, and stored for the long, cold Octobers, Novembers, Decembers, Januarys, and Februarys.

The Delamaters grew fewer types of vegetables than I do, and likely just one variety of each of those that they did grow. But they grew vegetables from across our eight families: cabbage, radishes, turnips, onions (red, yellow, and white), pole beans, peas, beets, spinach, lettuce, carrots, celery, parsnips, cucumbers, melons, squash, pumpkins, and potatoes.

Dinner (our lunch) was the main meal, composed of pork or fish with vegetables and bread. The vegetables were nearly always boiled. Hard apple cider was plentiful and, in that day, safer than the water.

The vitamin content of vegetables—a topic that I have probably overemphasized across these pages—was completely irrelevant to the Delamater family, as the first vitamins would not be discovered for another eighty years. Protein, antioxidants, and the like, too, were not yet part of the lexicon and were irrelevant to their eating. With this type of eating, and this extent of physical activity on the farm, overweight and obesity were virtually unheard of. So too were type 2 diabetes, hypertension, and some of our other diseases. Vegetarianism didn't really exist at the time, nor did it need to.

There was no such concept as local food for the Delamater family, as everything eaten was local, either from here on our land or bartered from the homesteads nearby. Likewise, there was no such idea as striving for seasonal eating, as what was eaten was determined entirely by the seasons. Nearly everything they ate was healthy: heirloom vegetables, whole foods from backyard gardens and barns, and local, pasture-raised meat. We can learn much about how to eat healthily by looking to how the Delamaters ate.

FROM HOME GARDENS TO HYDROGENATED OILS

The Delamater homestead was presumably a typical one. Food was local, meaning sourced almost completely on the property, and thus eating was always seasonal. Most everyone at the time, at least in rural areas, had gardens and produced their own eggs, milk, butter, vegetables, fruits, grains for breads, fresh meats, and cured meats. As markets and groceries became more common, some food items would be easier to just purchase, though they would have still been locally produced, and most of the household's food would still have come from the homestead.

The Delamater family's root cellar was more important than every appliance in my kitchen. Storing summer food for the winter months would advance further in 1858, when John Mason patented the Mason jar, and in 1884, when the Ball Brothers company started manufacturing glass jars for home canning, a process that peaked during World War II. The federal government encouraged home canning and gave guidance on numerous occasions to make the process safe. Rather than "putting down" vegetables in the root cellar, women were "putting up" vegetables by canning. Community canning centers opened so that grannies and their daughters and granddaughters could take their green beans, peaches, and the like for canning in a safe, shared facility with support staff. Freezing of homegrown vegetables obviously became common as well, as home freezers became increasingly available.

As transportation advanced, grocery stores became supersized, and employment patterns changed, the country shifted away from local and seasonal produce. Looking to the past—how Hannah, Cornelius, and the kids ate—has been helpful to me as I think about how a family can and did eat sustainably. But now we must look to the future and figure out how we're going to eat sustainably once again.

Where have all the gardens gone? Home gardens are uncommon compared to when Hannah and Cornelius lived. Where have all the community canneries gone? They are becoming, or have become, obsolete. The increasing availability of processed foods, like commercially canned vegetables, coincided with the decline in home canning. And with the advent of supermarkets and eighteen-wheelers came non-local, out-of-season produce, and, importantly, edible food-like substances, the foundation of our modern Western Diet. It's SAD: the Standard American Diet.

Edible food-like substances? That's Michael Pollan's clever term for ultra-processed foods. Edible? Yes. Food? No. The World Health Organization, among other health authorities, describes ultra-processed foods (which I'll now refer to as UPF) as "snacks, drinks, frozen meals, and many other product types formulated mostly or entirely from substances extracted from foods or derived from food constituents…made possible by the use of many types of additives, including those that imitate or enhance the sensory qualities of foods." That's a mouthful. They're "formulations of ingredients, mostly of exclusive industrial use"—"varieties of sugars (fructose, high-fructose corn syrup, 'fruit juice concentrates,' invert sugar, maltodextrin, dextrose, lactose), modified oils (hydrogenated or interesterified oils), and sources of protein (hydrolyzed proteins, soy protein isolate, gluten, casein, whey protein, and 'mechanically separated meats')"—"created by a series of industrial techniques and processes."

We're talking here about soft drinks, energy drinks, and fruit juice products; "sweet, fatty or salty packaged snacks; candies (confectionary); mass produced packaged breads and buns, cookies (biscuits), pastries, cakes and cake mixes; margarine and other spreads; sweetened breakfast 'cereals' and fruit yoghurts"; pre-prepared meats and cheeses; protein shakes; chicken nuggets, fish sticks, and the like; "sausages, burgers, hot dogs and other reconstituted meat products; powdered and packaged 'instant' soups, noodles, and desserts; baby formula; and many other types of product." These are things you can't make in your kitchen because you don't have the (industrial) ingredients in your pantry. Edible food-like substances. Edible? Yes. Food? No.

The current Western Diet (or SAD) relies heavily on UPF, largely pushing vegetables off the plate, and thus we have our current epidemic of obesity and food-related conditions like type 2 diabetes and cardiovascular disease. Additionally, this Western Diet is not good for our land and not good for the environment. But, as we all know, here we are.

The only way to get us out of this mess is to back our way out of it. More home gardens. More home canning, freezing, and curing. More meals made from scratch using regular ingredients and not industrial ones. And, when food is purchased, more local food. The backing out needs to be done by individuals in their homes, on their properties, returning, at least in part, to some level of homesteading, but it also needs to be done at the societal level, through advocacy and policy change.

It's not going to be easy or fast. Constructing the UPF mega-industry required great sophistication and took time, and deconstructing it will require our smarts and take time as well. We have to back our way out of it—our health depends on it.

FAKE HAMBURGERS WITH LAXATIVES

A recent advance in UPF is fake meat. I would have, just a few years ago, thought it to be beyond impossible what industry has now accomplished: "plant-based" meat alternatives. Again, edible food-like substances. Meat? No. Edible? Yes. Food? No. Read the ingredients. I don't know what things like cultured dextrose, methylcellulose, soy leghemoglobin, soy protein concentrate, sunflower lecithin, and the like are, and I don't have them in my pantry. The leghemoglobin has something to do with fermentation of genetically engineered yeast to get the bloody, meaty taste of hamburgers. The methylcellulose rings a bell from medical school, as it's a commonly used over-the-counter laxative. But in this case, it's being used to bulk up the patty rather than the poop. Aside from the exact industrial ingredients, creating this meatless meat is very sophisticated technology—high science, in fact. The fake meat is made in ultra-modern industrial laboratories, no cow pastures required.

In my opinion, if one just wants the experience of eating a burger, not craving the meat per se, then why not make a homemade veggie burger? Recipes commonly call for broccoli, onion, black beans, spinach, and carrot, among other ingredients sure to be in your pantry. Eat it with a leaf lettuce and a slice of juicy, ripe tomato, and that's seven families!

It's almost impossible to go beyond that! Roasted squash as a side makes it eight. No fake blood—or methylcellulose or other stool-bulking laxatives—are needed.

And in my opinion, if one so craves meat that one will eat industrial fake meat, then one should just eat meat. Ideally, local meet. And that's coming from a doctor who declared that bacon, ham, and sausage are bad and that we should stop eating them, a doctor who is advocating for a whole-foods, plant-predominant eating pattern. I have the same thoughts about vegan chicken nuggets and the like; it's simply replacing one UPF substance that contains chicken parts with another UPF substance without chicken parts. Just eat actual chicken parts. Ideally, from local chickens. Again, this is coming from someone who is really recommending a whole-foods, plant-predominant eating pattern.

As noted, if you do eat meat, for the sake of our environment, it should be local meat in small portions, not CAFO meat—in other words, the type of meat the Delamaters ate. And they ate meat in moderation.

BLUEBERRY MUFFINS WITH NO BLUEBERRIES

Do you ever want a blueberry muffin at breakfast instead of quiche and a salad? Some mornings I do. Here, I'm going to use blueberry muffins to make a point. The point could be made with thousands upon thousands of other edible food-like substances available in the grocery store. In fact, the vast majority of the food in grocery stores is UPF. This is the situation that we have to figure out how to back ourselves out of.

The moral of the story here is to make blueberry muffins with blueberries.

Edible-food-like-substance blueberry muffins are easy to make using one of the mixes in cardboard boxes in the middle isles of the grocery store. All you have to do is add an egg and milk. But here's what's in the mix: wheat flour and sugar (I have no issues with the ingredients list so far), animal shortening (lard, hydrogenated lard, tocopherols preservative, butylated hydroxytoluene preservative, citric acid preservative), dextrose, salt, baking soda, palm oil, sodium aluminum phosphate, monocalcium phosphate, fructose, food-starch modified, natural and artificial flavors (unspecified further, which is okay with the FDA), tricalcium phosphate, citric acid, Blue 2 Lake, Red 40 Lake, wheat starch, niacin, reduced iron, thiamine mononitrate, riboflavin, folic acid, and silicone dioxide. No blueberries. Zero. Zilch.

Those things that look like blueberries are not blueberries. They're concoctions of industrial ingredients meant to make us think they're blueberries. They're made in ultra-modern industrial laboratories, no blueberry bushes needed. According to the FDA, a color additive, as defined by federal regulation, is "any dye, pigment, or other substance" that can "impart color" to a "food, drug, or cosmetic"; color additives are "important components of many products, making them attractive, appealing, appetizing, and informative. Added color serves as a kind of code that allows us to identify products on sight, like candy flavors, medicine dosages, and left or right contact lenses." That is the federal government speaking. Those things that look like blueberries "impart color" and make the muffin "attractive, appealing, appetizing," while serving as "a kind of code that allows us to identify [these non-blueberry blueberry muffins] on sight."

Color additives, evidently, are classified by federal standards as "straight colors, lakes, and mixtures." Lakes—in this case, Blue 2 Lake and Red 40 Lake, which are needed to make the blueberry muffins "attractive, appealing, appetizing" with the fake blueberry concoctions—are made through chemical reactions with "aluminum cation as the precipitant and aluminum hydroxide as the substratum." I don't know what that means. Red 40 Lake is evidently used in food and cosmetics, and like Blue 2 Lake, is evidently made from coal tar or petroleum. I don't understand the industrial engineering that goes into making these industrial ingredients, but I do know that I would much rather wear Red 40 Lake makeup than eat fake blueberries. The blueberry muffins in restaurant chains are likely made with this same type of mix. It is not food. But it is edible, as is the cardboard box the mixture came in: Lots of fiber? Yes. Edible? Yes. Food? No. Even if all the ingredients in the cardboard box are completely benign from a health perspective, approved for human consumption by the federal government, and backed by science from the industries, the whole process is bad for our land and for the environment.

Why not just eat blueberry muffins with blueberries?

Blueberry muffins can be made from scratch, at home, like quiche can. You'll need flour and sugar. And then, rather than all those industrial substances, you'll need salt, baking powder, and some oil. And the egg and the milk. Oh, and blueberries. Fresh in the early summer, or those frozen during the early summer for the rest of the year. Eight ingredients, not twenty-five, and no cardboard.

EATING LOCAL AND COOKING FROM SCRATCH

In my view—biased for sure as a home gardener, CSA operator, and farmers market vendor—the most important step forward is to eat local to the largest extent possible, ingredients grown as close to your kitchen as is feasible. The best-case scenario is to grow as much of your own food as possible. I know that sounds radical and perhaps even alarmist, but if you can grow your own lettuce in the spring, your own tomatoes in the summer, your own cabbage in the fall, and so on, you will benefit mentally and physically. You'll experience pride and a sense of accomplishment, which is good for your mental health, and you'll eat the healthiest food possible, obviously good for your physical health. And it will have been good for the environment and thus for all of us. People had gardens. We can have them again.

When a garden is infeasible for whatever reason, the next best option is to rely on one or more local farmers to provide as much of your food as possible. A great way to connect with a local farmer is to join a CSA. It's an ideal business model for the small farmer, and it connects you directly with the grower. He or she becomes, in effect, *your* farmer. Alternatively, or in addition, farmers markets offer a huge array of interesting and delicious produce, and, again, you can interact with the very people who labored to produce it. Since eating local means eating seasonal, some of us are going to have to get used to no fresh tomatoes in the winter months, along with many other adjustments.

We can use local produce to make our own processed foods, substituting them for UPF. When making jam using local fruit, we won't add GMO-based high-fructose corn syrup, or corn syrup, or artificial coloring, or "natural flavorings," which are actually industrial concoctions. It's probably just going to contain fruit, a tart green apple for pectin, and sugar. Make your own salsa, marina, pesto, and the like. It's also possible to make your own ketchup, which will not contain industrial GMO-based corn substances, and you can even make your own mayonnaise, free of industrial GMO-based soy substances. We're going to have to do these things, turning back to how they used to eat in this old stone house, in order to survive. Eating UPF, in my opinion, is not only deadly but most definitely not sustainable.

EATING TWO HUNDRED YEARS FROM NOW

I wonder what our meals will look like two hundred years from now. Surely, someone, a couple or a family, will be eating meals in the dining room of this old stone house. What will they be eating? Presumably, vegetables, fruits, grains, dairy, eggs, and meats not dissimilar to what we eat, likely with a number of new varieties of vegetables, thanks to Mother Nature's gift of natural cross-pollination and our smarts at controlled cross-pollination. I hope that they will be eating less—much less, not more—ultra-processed edible food-like substances.

Rather than industrial ingredients with adverse impacts on our soil, our water, and our health, we will need to backtrack so that eating looks more similar to how the Delamater family ate, at least in some respects—not coals underneath Dutch ovens in an open hearth, but also not cardboard boxes of unnatural industrial ingredients that include blue things designed to make us think they're blueberries. More of us will need to plant blueberry bushes, not on an industrial scale requiring repeated drenching of animal-killing chemicals, but the kind that I grow, and the kind that you can grow. They are simply bushes, and they require very limited specific horticultural skill—perhaps not even green thumbs.

How we eat meat most definitely must change. Ongoing deforestation for more CAFOs is not the way to go, obviously. Ongoing extensive use of herbicides on fields where GMO herbicide-tolerant commodity crops are grown for those animals is obviously not the way to go. They want to eat grass and grains and weeds, not GMO corn.

We must embrace sustainability in our food supply. We owe it to our future generations. We need actual sustainability—way fewer inputs, fewer externalities, minimal industrial processing, markedly reduced food travel distances.

Homo sapiens, the genus and species about which I have heretofore spoken too little despite my fondness for them, was able to eat sustainably before. The Delamaters surely did. Now, in the Anthropocene, we must figure out how to once again eat sustainably. If our species was able to figure out, so sophisticatedly, how to eat in a way that is definitely not sustainable, then we can figure out actual sustainability. Not only can we do it, but we must.

Free Health Advice from a Doctor and Farmer

THESE RECOMMENDATIONS, based on everything I've learned as a doctor and farmer, have improved my own health. I hope that they will be helpful and healthful to you as well.

1. *Get smart about vegetables.*

2. *Strive for eight on my plate.*

3. *Nurture a relationship with each vegetable mentioned in this book.* Become acquainted with each one, especially those most underappreciated and those that can be deemed superfoods (like the Brassicas, the Legumes, and the Chenopods). Try each vegetable mentioned in this book at least three times, using three different preparation methods or recipes, before deciding against any given vegetable. In doing so, identify your vegetable addictions.

4. *Get to know one or more small local farms.* They need our support.

5. *Eat local and organic to the largest extent possible.* Join a local CSA, or buy produce from local farmers market as much as possible. Shop in small, local grocery stores that buy from local farmers. Eat at "farm to table" restaurants that source products from local farmers. These purchasing practices not only support

the goal of sustainable farming practices but also, importantly, support small, local farms in terms of financial sustainability. Read about the local food movement, the one-hundred-mile diet, the slow food movement, sustainable agriculture, food justice, and food sovereignty. In addition to local, eat organic produce when possible. The organic label—despite some lingering problems with the rules, regulations, and allowances behind the label—disallows GMO seeds, and organic produce is "clean" without pesticide residues.

6. *Even better than just local, plant a garden—that's super local.* Grow all eight families. Grow too much in order to try freezing and canning vegetables. And grow too much in order to share the bounties with family, friends, and neighbors. It will delight them. It can strengthen your relationships with them. As part of the garden, plant a few blueberry bushes. And consider currants. Gardens are easy, even with the smallest patch of land, and can bring about not just vegetables but improved emotional well-being. Gardens also provide (require) physical activity, which is second only to a healthy way of eating as the one prescription from which we would all benefit most. Gardens also teach us about vegetables and fruits (and flowers!), deepening our understanding and appreciation for these very generous genera and species.

7. *Grow some portion of your own food.* If not a garden, it might simply be pea and sunflower shoots in

the kitchen, a cherry tomato plant surrounded by parsley and basil in a planter on the balcony, one small raised bed in the backyard, or interplanting a flower bed with kale and Swiss chard. Everyone should grow some portion—no matter how small—of their own food, the more the better. I offer consultations on how to grow some of your own food or build a garden. Some other farmers do, too.

8. *Read Deborah Madison's cookbook: Vegetable Literacy: Cooking and Gardening with Twelve Families from the Edible Plant Kingdom, with over 300 Deliciously Simple Recipes.* She's a renowned chef who knows all about the eight families (and four others) by having grown them and having spent a career perfecting delicious recipes for every vegetable imaginable. It's a cookbook with so many mouth-watering veggie recipes, but it's also a delight to read from cover to cover. There are many other outstanding vegetable cookbooks out there, including Steven Satterfield's *Vegetable Revelations: Inspiration for Produce-Forward Cooking* and Laura Sorkin's *Vegetables: The Ultimate Cookbook Featuring 300+ Delicious Plant-Based Recipes,* to name just two.

9. *Set and achieve goals pertaining to a regular, healthy way of eating; avoid going on a "diet."* Diets tend to be short-lived, with results equally transient. A consistent, healthy way of eating, despite some imperfections and occasional splurges, promotes improved health in the long term.

10. *Replace white bread with brown bread.* Ideally, the brown bread will have lots of visible seeds. Brown pasta is better than white pasta, brown rice better than white. For all of these starches, brown is better than white.

11. *Minimize saturated fat and maximize fiber.* This might be my most important recommendation for health promotion and disease prevention. It means leaning toward plant-derived foods like vegetables, fruits, nuts, seeds, and grains and leaning away from animal-derived foods like meat, cheese, and butter.

12. *Make hummus. Make pesto. Make gazpacho.* They are so easy and so delicious.

13. *Figure out which vegetables you most enjoy for breakfast.* Yes, add some vegetables to breakfast; potatoes don't count (unless you grew them).

14. *Consider two uses for vegetable scraps from the kitchen: vegetable stock and/or composting.* Collard stems. Leek tops. Pea pods. Wilted Swiss chard. Outer radicchio leaves. Bolted dill. Squash rinds. Eggplant bottoms. You name it. They make a great stock, and they create very rich soil.

15. *If you eat meat, replace some of it with other complete proteins.* These include, among others, beans with rice, hummus and pita, and single-ingredient peanut butter on whole-grain bread. Eat edamame and tofu. Try quinoa and amaranth.

16. *If you eat meat entrées, replace some of them with vegetable entrées.* These might include a loaded veg-

etable pizza, pasta primavera, eggplant "meatballs," and veggie "burgers" (those made with vegetables, not fake meat).

17. *If you eat meat, eat local, and meet the meat before you eat the meat.* Visit a local farm and meet the cow or pig or chicken that will be turned into meat for you. I know that sounds radical, or perhaps seemingly impossible, but this is how the Delamaters ate, and for many of us, we can get our meat from local farms where we can get to know the farmer as well as what they grow, plants and animals alike. Meet the chickens that produce your eggs to see how they live. And meet the cows that make your milk and other dairy products. Meeting the animals will make both kids and adults feel happy; it is good for our mental health. If we leave not feeling happy, then eating those products is not good for our health. If we are prohibited from visiting the CAFOs where most eggs and meat are produced, or are not happy after the visit, then we shouldn't eat products from those facilities.

18. *Don't eat processed meats.* These include, among others, bacon, ham, sausage, salami, cold cuts, and hot dogs. A once-a-season splurge on a dog or a brat at a home game might well be acceptable.

19. *Packaged processed food (which may be healthy or unhealthy) and ultra-processed food (which, by definition, is most likely unhealthy) are required to have a Nutrition Facts label—read it.* The label is very informative, giving servings per container, serving

size, calories per serving, saturated fat, cholesterol, sodium, total sugars including added sugars, and more. Foods without a Nutrition Facts label (read: vegetables and fruits) are the healthiest.

20. *Also read the list of ingredients.* If included in the list are any ingredients that you either cannot pronounce or that you do not have in your pantry, do not eat it or drink it. Also, as we should all know by now, be weary of any foods making health claims— that often means they are unhealthy.

21. *Be intentional when ordering prepared meals to be eaten out or in restaurants.* These meals are not required to have Nutrition Facts labels; that does not mean, however, that they do not contain ultra-processed foods. They also often are high in added sugars, added salt, and unhealthy fats.

22. *Recognize the complex relationship between GMOs, UPF, CAFOs, poor health, chronic disease, and environmental degradation.* Avoid GMOs, UPF, and CAFO meat and eggs. Steer clear of steer, especially steer and other livestock from CAFOs. They eat GMOs, though they shouldn't, like we shouldn't. You can assume that meat and eggs are from CAFOs unless it is very clearly specified (for example, from a named local farm) on the packaging or the menu. The best way to not eat GMOs is to avoid UPF. The industrial food complex and governmental policy are currently structured to encourage commodity crop farmers to grow GMOs and use pesticides, and for small livestock farms to supply or become part

of the CAFO system. As noted, small farms need our support.

23. *Speaking of avoiding UPF, read Michael Pollan's brilliant little book Food Rules: An Eater's Manual.* Though dozens of fun and funny rules are curated in it, his overarching rule is given in just seven words: "Eat Food. Mostly Plants. Not Too Much." The first idea is to eat food and not food-like substances— the kind of blueberry muffins that you can make from scratch, rather than the kind that the massive industrial food complex wants us to eat. Regarding the second ("Mostly Plants"), getting smart about vegetables and striving for eight on my plate is the way to go.

24. *Shake spices more than salt.*

25. *Drink from the tap.* Bottled water is an unusual and unnecessary industrial invention.

26. *Replace sugar-sweetened beverages with tap water flavored with whole fruits.* Use whole fruits like cucumbers, ground cherries, blueberries, lemons, and the like.

27. *Your doctor knows your BMI—you should know it too.* If thirty or more, ask your doctor for a referral to a registered dietitian nutritionist or a lifestyle medicine clinician. I offer consultations around lifestyle for health, as do so many other lifestyle medicine experts.

28. *Gradual weight gain means that energy (calories) IN is exceeding energy (calories) OUT.* While it's a very

basic equation representing very complex metabolic physiology, gradual weight gain indicates that more calories are being eaten (fats, proteins, and carbohydrates) than are being burned (through everyday physiological functions, all forms of movement and physical activity, and exercise). Stopping weight gain, or starting weight loss, requires taking in fewer calories and/or burning more.

29. *Make your own vitamin D while vigorously gardening.* But also use sun protection.

30. *Embrace other health-promoting and disease-preventing lifestyle changes.* This vegetable journey has been about embracing a whole-foods, plant-predominant eating pattern by getting smart about vegetables. As a lifestyle medicine physician, I encourage you to also embrace the other pillars of my profession to help you prevent, or even reverse, chronic diseases like type 2 diabetes, hypertension, and cardiovascular disease. These proven lifestyle interventions include getting enough physical activity, having restful and restorative sleep, using strategies for successful stress management, avoiding risky substance use, and ensuring that we have positive social connections, such as those in the garden, those around the kitchen countertop, and those at the table.

EPILOGUE

This Year's Farm

I'VE BEEN WRITING IN MY OLD STONE HOUSE FOR THREE WINTERS NOW—daydreaming and scribbling thoughts about delicious summertime vegetables that I'll be growing soon and savoring soon thereafter. Others who lived in this old stone house before me had similar wintertime daydreams about spring arriving and summertime growing.

This story ends as this winter is ending. March arrives tomorrow, and the garlic will soon appear from its slumber. I can now feel myself awakening from a haze, with a nearly electrical-feeling energy returning to my body and my mind. I'll soon have a rush of renewed motivation and ambition, fully awake, taking part in the push of spring, feeling the renewal of life. In ten days, it'll be time to prune the red currants and begin the cycle of currant bush propagation for next year's farm customers, Granny with me at each step of the way, helping me decide where to make the cuts and how many one-year-old, two-year-old, and three-year-old canes to let remain. Brown sticks will soon bear leaves, then flowers, then fruit. Spring is arriving, and soon a summer rich with beautiful, delicious, and nutritious vegetables.

The farm is different each year, and this year it will be quite unique. Instead of the CSA and farmers markets, I'll spend the season nerding out over winter squash, fourteen varieties of *Cucurbita*, inspired in part by Amy across the river. Maybe my autumn frost butternut and my burgess buttercup will be served in the dining rooms of hundreds—or thousands if the harvest is grand—of Ulster County residents this fall. And I'll geek out with perhaps the four most underappreciated—at least in the United States—of all the vegetables: the chicories, *Cichorium endivia* (escarole and frisée) and *Cichorium intybus* (catalogna and radicchio). I'll grow every variety I can find, many dozens; I'll study them through fieldwork on the farm and then in Italy; and I'll write about them next winter, with a lofty goal of popularizing the chicory vegetables in America.

I'll grow as much of this produce within my tight dimensions as I possibly can, and I'll delight the neighbors with the tart red currants that Granny and I have grown, with gooseberries, with black raspberries, with pea shoots, with Valentine and the many other cherry tomato varieties, and, if my trials are a success, with big boxes of radicchio and eventually bushels of winter squash.

My relationships with vegetables will continue to evolve on this year's farm. I'm going to try to grow spinach, once again, like every year. Maybe I'll take an online class or watch a YouTube video. I'm going to make space for a bed of brussels sprouts and a bed of parsnips, even though they take so long. I'm going to reevaluate my ambivalent relationship with several vegetables that I've perhaps inappropriately called "strange," like artichokes and salsify—striving to overcome my ambivalence and hopefully achieving a more satisfying, stable, long-term, and healthy relationship with them and several others. I'm going to figure out a system to grow watercress. And one to force select radicchios into Belgian endive.

On this year's farm, I'm going to commit myself to pulling more weeds and to eating more weeds—garlic mustard from the Brassicas, wild garlic and wild onions from the Alliums, lamb's quarters and pigweed from the Chenopods, purslane, and more.

I'm going to try to eat even more pizza for dinner. Loaded with my veggies, of course.

I'm going to make red currant jam, and my Granny Essie Mae will be so proud of what we together have done. I'm going to make red raspberry jam to eat right here in this old stone house, and Granny Hannah will be so proud of what we together have done. I'm going to craft delicious blueberry muffins, from scratch, with blueberries, lots of blueberries, my own blueberries.

This old stone house, this land, this little under-an-acre farm, these many thousands of plants from seedlings to harvest, these unexpected midlife tons of produce, this learning have been among the greatest joys, and perhaps the most meaningful journey, of my life. We'll stay here longer than Ira Lambert did, though not nearly as long as Hannah or Yancey.

I'll have new journeys. Maybe I'll move south and learn to grow bananas and mangos. Always, though, my heart, my joy, my health will be tied to this piece of land, this little farm that I built elbow-to-elbow with Sheri and Sam, and Anthony, Paul, Kristopher, Hannah, Ian, Christina, and Chad—with the help of Charlie's plow, the encouragement and sunset toasts of Peter and Ande across the road, and the loyalty of my farm members and farmers market customers—growing these eight families that I have rejoiced in savoring and sharing, here on Yancey's property, the Delamater homestead, this land of the Lenape.

Acknowledgments

OUTSIDE, ON THE FARM, I owe gratitude to everyone who helped me build this little vegetable operation. Anthony. Paul. Kristopher. Hannah. Ian. Christina. Chad. But especially Sheri and Sam—two serious veggie nerds, or more accurately, vegetable bon vivants. In growing with you, so many pairs of green thumbs, I hope that we have helped others grow stronger, healthier, and happier. Additionally, the work could not have been done without the support of our farm share members and farmers market customers—thank you for trusting me as your veggie farmer.

INSIDE, AT THE DESK, I am grateful to Coleen, my agent; Adriana and Aleigha, my editors; and Gretchen, my publisher. In your working with me, a nerdy farmer who goes on about radicchio aspirations, I hope that we too will help others be stronger, healthier, and happier. I've got a butternut squash for each of you when I see you next. And, importantly, this work would not have been done without the hope for many readers, who I thank in advance for considering the ideas I share on savoring all of these vegetables.

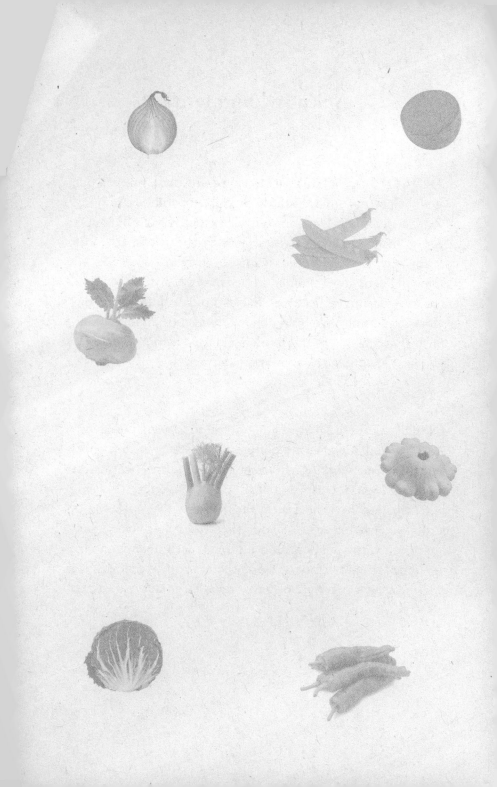